GLOW

THE DERMATOLOGIST'S GUIDE TO A WHOLE FOODS YOUNGER SKIN DIET

RAJANI KATTA M.D.

PUBLISHED BY

MD2B

HOUSTON, TEXAS

www.MD2B.net

Glow: The Dermatologist's Guide to a Whole Foods Younger Skin Diet is published by MD2B, PO Box 300988, Houston, TX 77230-0988.

www.MD2B.net

NOTICE: The recommendations in this book are based on a thorough review of research performed in the field, and are presented to help readers make informed decisions about their health. Readers should not view this information as a substitute for any treatment recommended by their physician. Before beginning a new exercise or diet program, it is the reader's responsibility to discuss their plans with their personal physician and obtain approval.

The author and publisher disclaim any personal liability, either directly or indirectly, for advice or information presented within. The author and publisher have used care and diligence in the preparation of this book. Every effort has been made to ensure the accuracy and completeness of information contained within this book. No responsibility is assumed for errors, inaccuracies, omissions, or any false or misleading implication that may arise due to the text.

Please note that any mention of specific companies, organizations, or authorities in this book should not be viewed as an endorsement by either the author or the publisher.

Recipes by Rajani Katta and Swarajyalaxmi Katta
Book Design by Shaan Desai and Jasmine Nguyen with formatting assistance by Samir Desai and Krishna Sigireddi
Research Assistants: Teja Desai, Sophia Huang, Jasmine Nguyen, Girija Shan, Michelle Zhong
Cover Photo by Suman Mangu
Photos (online): Rajani Katta, Shaan Desai, Anna Katta, Praveen Katta, Sharon Lunbeck, Denise Metry MD

Printed in the United States of America

ISBN # 9781937978099

DEDICATION

We often don't realize the power of a kind word shared at the right time. I am blessed to have wonderful, uplifting, supportive friends and family, and to them I say thank you for the kind words and support over many years.

And to the many individuals out there who are so kind and helpful and giving of their time and resources, even to perfect strangers: thank you.

ABOUT THE AUTHOR

A nationally recognized expert in dermatology and allergic contact dermatitis, Dr. Rajani Katta has extensively researched how diet can affect the skin and the body's overall health. Her advice on skin care and diet has been published in many magazines and newspapers, including the Oprah Magazine, Prevention, Glamour, Good Housekeeping, Men's Health, and the Dr. Oz magazine. She has been interviewed as a dermatology expert on the ABC, CBS, Fox, and NBC networks, as well as NPR and multiple radio stations.

Committed to furthering the understanding of skin disease, Dr. Katta has authored over 70 scientific articles and chapters in prestigious publications, including the *Journal of the American Academy of Dermatology*. She has also been honored to serve on the Review Panels for the *Archives of Dermatology*, *Journal of the American Academy of Dermatology*, and *American Family Physician*. She is an accomplished speaker, and has lectured frequently at national meetings of the American Academy of Dermatology and the American Contact Dermatitis Society. She has also spoken at such institutions as the University of Chicago, Northwestern University, and the University of Southern California.

Dr. Katta served as Professor of Dermatology at the Baylor College of Medicine for over 17 years, during which time she oversaw the dermatology basic science education of over 2,500 medical students. She is an award-winning educator, and the author of 6 highly acclaimed books on medical student success. She continues to mentor and teach the next generation of physicians as a clinical faculty member at both the Baylor College of Medicine and the McGovern Medical School at the University of Texas Houston.

For her dedication to excellence in patient care, teaching, and research, she has been the recipient of multiple awards, including the Fulbright and Jaworski Faculty Excellence Award. She is a member of the Alpha Omega Alpha Honor Medical Society and Phi Beta Kappa, and has been named to the Texas Super Doctors® list.

SECTION ONE
YOUTHFUL SKIN

SECTION TWO
WHAT TO EAT

SECTION THREE
DIET AND DERMATOLOGY

SECTION FOUR
RECIPES

Section 1

YOUTHFUL SKIN

CHAPTER 1
INTRODUCTION

Over the 20 years that I've been caring for patients as a dermatologist, I've been asked a lot of questions about how to prevent aging skin. Here are a few that I've been asked by patients and friends (*names changed):

- Mrs. Riley is in her early 50s, and she's started to notice a softening of her jawline. She hasn't developed jowls yet (those loose folds of skin hanging off the jawline), but she's worried she's heading that way.

- Celeste is in her 20s, and her friends have all started getting serious about sunblock and anti-aging skin care regimens. One of her friends keeps telling her that she needs to start getting regular injections of Botox as part of an anti-aging skin regimen. She has her doubts about that, but she's wondering if there's anything else she should be doing to take care of her skin.

- Mr. Henderson is in his 70s, and he's here because of his grandchildren. His young grandson keeps asking about the dark purple spots on his forearms. He knows these are due to fragile skin which leads him to bruise easily, but he's worried this will get worse.

- Mrs. Boyd has always had a very smooth, youthful complexion, but now that she's in her late 30s she's noticing crow's feet: fine lines at the corners of her eyes. She's using a good anti-aging skin care regimen, and she's very careful to use sunscreen and large sunglasses when outdoors. She's wondering what else she can do to slow down the formation of new wrinkles.

- Laura is in her mid-40s, and she's noticed many more dark spots and freckles on her face in the last 5 years. They're much more prominent now than ever before, and she's having a hard time covering them with concealer. She knows that a lot of this is her beach exposure catching up to her years later, and she's planning to have laser treatment to lighten the dark spots. She wants to know what else she can do to prevent more dark spots.

The skin concerns that Mr. Henderson, Mrs. Boyd, and Laura describe may all sound different, but they all share one important point.

They're all common signs of aging skin.

————————————————

In medical circles we use certain terms to describe these concerns. Loss of elasticity. Fine lines and wrinkles. Solar lentigos (dark spots).

These are all skin changes that become increasingly common with age, and it might seem as though you're powerless to combat them. But the reality is that you can do much more than you realize.

What Would I Tell Each And Every One Of These Patients?

- I would tell them that you have the power to prevent further damage.
- I would tell them that you have the power to promote the skin's ability to regenerate.
- And I would tell them that this power, exercised in small ways every single day, can add up to big benefits.

Where does this power come from?

It comes from the choices that we make every day – including the foods that we eat.

The right foods play an important role in this process. Along with consistent sun protection and the right products or procedures, the promise of more youthful skin is more attainable than ever.

The Right Foods Provide Power: The Power to Prevent Skin Damage and The Power to Promote Skin Regeneration

Your skin is the largest organ of your body, and it is amazing. It protects you from extremes of temperature, from UV radiation, from infection, and more.

And it has a remarkable ability to regenerate. Think about the last time you had a paper cut. (That painful one. On the tip of your thumb. The one that made you wince every time you turned the page.)

Just two days later, and it was gone. Completely healed. On its own.

Healed so completely, in fact, that it was as though it had never been there at all.

That's what your skin can do: it has amazing abilities to repair and regenerate.

The right foods can support and supercharge those systems.

What Can The Right Foods Do For Your Skin? They Can:

QUENCH FREE RADICALS Your skin is under siege. Every minute of every day. Which is why your skin has so many built-in defense and repair mechanisms.

We know that ultraviolet (UV) radiation ages the skin. And the more that hits the skin, the more damage that results. You might see this as a sunburn. But even without a visible burn, that radiation produces free radicals and "burns" your skin on a cellular level, with damage to DNA, collagen fibers, elastic fibers, and more.

Antioxidants act to quench that damage. Some are naturally found in your skin, but they're constantly being used up. That's why the antioxidants in your food are so important: they provide a constant, renewable source of quenching antioxidants.

BLOCK SCISSOR ENZYMES UV radiation also damages the skin by increasing levels of "scissor" enzymes. These enzymes, including collagenase and elastase, start snapping away at the collagen fibers and elastic fibers that maintain youthful, resilient skin. The right foods prevent the activation of scissor enzymes.

ACTIVATE DNA REPAIR SYSTEMS When DNA damage does occur, your body springs into action to repair that damage. The right foods work to activate this system.

STRENGTHEN THE SKIN BARRIER The right foods can also help regenerate the skin barrier. Your skin barrier has two main functions: keep moisture in and keep irritants out (along with microbes, allergens, and toxins). As you age, that barrier doesn't work as well. The right foods, including the right fats, can help strengthen that skin barrier.

PROMOTE THE GROWTH OF GOOD MICROBES THAT STRENGTHEN THE SKIN BARRIER A healthy gut can also strengthen the skin barrier. Certain "good" microbes that live in your gastrointestinal tract can produce substances that actually strengthen the skin barrier. The right foods can promote the growth of these good microbes.

The Research That Can Help You Take Action

Over the next 200+ pages, you'll learn more. More about the forces that threaten your skin, and more about the research on how to combat those forces. You'll especially learn more about the foods that play such an important role in maintaining youthful skin.

While you'll learn about the research, this book is focused on action. You'll learn about the forces that work to damage your skin, and you'll learn about the foods that work to combat those forces. I call these skin saving foods, and in Section 4 you'll find recipes that make use of these powerful foods.

If you'd like to read more about the research, my website SkinAndDiet.com contains more information. You'll find links to the articles that I've written for a medical audience, published in peer reviewed medical journals. These articles cite the work of many amazing researchers in the field.

In the chapters to come, you'll learn how to translate this research into action to achieve youthful, glowing skin.

CHAPTER 2
A HOLISTIC APPROACH

I was on a hillside trail in Arizona, just starting a hike, when I saw a very striking woman coming down the path towards me. She was laughing and flushed and she looked exhilarated. She was absolutely luminous.

My guess was that she was in her 70s, and her face did have wrinkles. The thing is, she was just so full of life that the wrinkles barely registered; what really struck me was how youthful and radiant she looked.

With modern technology and skin care advances, there's a lot that can be done to address skin care concerns. But that inner glow of health and vitality: to achieve that requires more than makeup and skin care. That's why I talk about a holistic approach to youthful, healthy skin.

If your diet were a pill, the ads would call it:

> *The Safe, Inexpensive, and Natural*
> *Antioxidant and Anti-Inflammatory*
> *Approach to Glowing, Youthful*
> *Skin!*

In the following pages, you'll learn a lot more about the research behind that statement supporting the role of diet in healthy skin. Notice that word "role". It's important to realize that diet has to be used along with other treatments and approaches for the best effects. As in so much of medicine, it's not about one single factor. You really have to think about health, and healthy skin, in a holistic way.

A Holistic Approach to Youthful, Healthy Skin

The recommended approach to youthful skin: Prevent, Promote, and Polish.

♦ **PREVENT** skin damage by protecting against UV radiation, pollution, advanced glycation end products, and other threats.

♦ **PROMOTE** skin health and skin regeneration by promoting high antioxidant levels, high anti-inflammatory activity, and good gut microbes.

♦ **POLISH** your skin's appearance by using the right skin care products, along with the right, carefully selected procedures when needed.

For Youthful, Healthy Skin

You need a holistic approach. It's not just about the right cream or the right procedure, although that may be part of it. A holistic approach means that you're looking at the whole picture. There are a number of factors that impact the health of your skin, and they're interconnected. To start with, you need to protect your skin on the outside from UV radiation and other threats. You also need to promote healthy skin by providing high levels of nutrients and promoting skin repair.

When it comes to promoting youthful, healthy skin, there are no quick fixes. There ARE quick fixes when it comes to repairing skin damage (technology is amazing). But promoting healthy skin requires taking small, consistent actions. To prevent sun damage, you have to protect yourself from UV radiation every single day. To promote youthful skin, you need to replete the nutrients in your skin every day.

Eating for youthful, healthy skin means focusing on your overall eating pattern. No one supplement, and no one food, is ever going to be as powerful as the combination of nutrients in a balanced, varied, nutrient-rich diet. That means a focus on a powerful, nutrient-rich, whole foods diet.

Eating for healthy skin means eating for health. The recommendations in the following chapters are the same as those recommended for the prevention of heart disease, hypertension, and Alzheimer's. That makes sense, because the health of our skin is so closely intertwined with our overall health. This fact is one of the main reasons I wanted to write this book. Eating more vegetables is one of the keys to fighting off some of the biggest threats to our nation's health, including diabetes, hypertension, and heart disease. The fact that vegetables and a whole foods diet promote glowing, younger skin gives you one more reason to eat more.

CHAPTER 3
THE SIGNS OF SKIN AGING

The signs of skin aging: they've been recognized (and worried over) for centuries.

The ancient Egyptians placed a great emphasis on skin preservation, in this life as well as the afterlife. Egyptian women traveled with makeup boxes containing their cosmetics and beauty tools. This care and concern extended to the afterlife: archaeological evidence has found that skin care products and tools were commonly placed in the tombs of the dead.

Just as in modern times, the ancient Egyptians were fighting the signs of skin aging:

THE SIGNS OF SKIN AGING

1. Fine lines and wrinkles. While some are due to aging itself, a major factor in the development of wrinkles is the amount of UV radiation that reaches your skin and damages the collagen and elastic fibers in the skin.

2. Sagging. Think about an elderly person with jowls, and how that contrasts with the firm jawline of a 20-year-old. That's due to collagen damage: accumulated collagen damage over a number of years weakens the supportive framework of your skin.

3. Loss of elasticity. Someone in their 20s has tight, taut skin that bounces back when you pinch it. As you age, your skin loses that ability to bounce back.

4. Atrophy. Your skin can become more fragile as you age. Many of my elderly patients describe frequent bruising on their forearms. They'll tell me that all it takes is a bump against the wall. This is because our skin thins as we age, which is known as skin atrophy. Sun exposure speeds up this process by damaging collagen.

5. Pigment changes. As we age, we accumulate a lot more freckles and dark spots. The medical term for one type of dark spot is solar lentigos. I call these sun spots, because they're due to a lifetime of UV exposure finally catching up to us.

6. Changes in skin texture. As you age, your skin often becomes more rough and dry. That's because your skin just doesn't hold onto moisture as well. And it doesn't matter how many glasses of water you drink--the loss of natural oils in our skin predisposes us to dry, rough skin as we age.

7. Loss of radiance and changes in microvasculature. Microvasculature is the medical term for the small blood vessels in our skin. Some people report that their skin looks more "sallow" as they age, meaning that they no longer have that healthy glow or radiance of youthful skin. It's believed that some of that is due to less blood flow through the tiny blood vessels that supply your skin.

Just as in ancient Egypt, this emphasis on preserving youthful skin was present in many of the advanced ancient civilizations, from China to the Middle East to India. Ayurvedic medicine, one of the most ancient medical traditions, had extensive descriptions of skin care techniques.

Practiced in India and other South Asian countries, ancient Ayurvedic texts describe skin care products (oils, powders, herbal waters) as well as ingested treatments. It's been reported that the ancient texts described over 200 herbs, minerals, and fats to maintain the health and beauty of the skin.

Their rationale for use centered around principles of anti-aging activity that we recognize today. In fact, many of the skin saving foods we recommend today target the same exact areas: cell regeneration, radiance, anti-inflammatory properties, and others.

Modern scientific research techniques have uncovered properties which may explain why these foods and herbs were considered so helpful. In one study, for example, the fruit Indian gooseberry [Phyllanthus emblica or amla] increased the activity of telomerase in the body, an enzyme with potential anti-aging properties.

Research has now shown that many different foods and nutrients can successfully target different cellular pathways.

Which means that a number of different foods can help you maintain youthful, luminous skin. The following table contains just a few examples of these foods.

THE RIGHT FOODS CAN COMBAT
THE VISIBLE SIGNS OF SKIN AGING

Fine Lines and Wrinkles	Foods rich in antioxidants can limit the collagen damage caused by free radicals: tomatoes (lycopene), berries (polyphenols), turmeric (curcumin), green tea (catechins)
Sagging	Advanced glycation end products (known as AGEs) can cause serious damage to collagen. These compounds are formed when sugar in your system bonds with proteins in your body, and they're a major cause of wrinkling and sagging. Foods that limit rapid, sharp spikes in blood sugar levels may help limit sugar sag.

- High fiber foods ensure steady blood sugar levels: vegetables
- Power carbs, naturally rich in fiber and protein, limit rapid rises in blood sugar levels: lentils, beans, whole grains
- Some herbs and spices may help stabilize blood sugar levels: cinnamon, fenugreek, garlic, ginger, onions, turmeric
- Healthy proteins can balance out carbs to limit sugar spikes: beans, lentils, tofu, eggs, salmon, shrimp
- Certain phytonutrients (which are beneficial compounds in plant foods), including luteolin, quercetin, and rutin, have been shown to fight the process of glycation: apples, asparagus, cauliflower, figs, onions

Loss of Elasticity	• Research indicates that some foods are able to block the activity of the scissor enzyme elastase. Elastase is triggered by UV radiation and acts to degrade the elastic fibers in the skin: ginger, white tea, pomegranate • Higher intake of MUFAs (monounsaturated fatty acids) has been linked to more skin elasticity: olive oil
Atrophy and Skin Fragility	Thinning of the skin occurs naturally with age, but is accelerated by UV radiation and other factors that cause collagen damage. • Vitamin C is an essential cofactor in collagen synthesis: broccoli, cauliflower, red peppers, citrus • Certain polyphenol phytonutrients, including apigenin and luteolin, inhibit the activity of collagenase, an enzyme that degrades collagen: artichokes, celery, basil, cilantro, parsley, thyme • Certain spices and herbs act to inhibit the production of collagen-damaging AGEs: cinnamon, cloves, oregano, allspice
Pigment Changes	Foods that limit the damage caused by UV exposure can limit the signs of photoaging, which includes freckling and solar lentigos. • Foods demonstrated in human research studies to limit the skin damage caused by UV radiation: tomatoes, green tea, cocoa flavanols, pomegranate • Foods rich in polyphenol phytonutrients: In one study, patients reporting higher intake had lower scores of UV-related pigmented spots

Texture Changes	Aging skin naturally exhibits a loss of natural oils and an increase in moisture loss.

- Foods rich in omega-3 fatty acids have been shown to reduce skin roughness and improve skin hydration: ground flaxseeds, walnuts, fatty fish such as salmon and sardines
- Foods rich in prebiotic fiber promote the growth of good gut microbes, which aid the function of the skin barrier: legumes, onions, garlic, asparagus, artichokes, oats
- Foods rich in live, active cultures of good microbes (probiotics) may improve skin barrier recovery: yogurt, miso, sauerkraut, kimchi, kefir, some vinegars, some pickled vegetables

Radiance	

- Foods rich in polyphenol phytonutrients may improve blood flow through the small blood vessels that supply the skin: grapes, berries, black beans
- In studies of human volunteers, higher levels of carotenoids in the skin impart a healthy glow: carrots, sweet potatoes, apricots, butternut squash

CHAPTER 4
THE KEYS TO EATING FOR MORE YOUTHFUL, HEALTHY SKIN

The 3 keys to eating for youthful skin:

1. Eat Power: Eat foods that provide powerful nutrients.

2. Stop Sugar Spikes: Elevations in blood sugar levels (sugar spikes) lead your body to produce AGEs (advanced glycation end products). These "sticky" compounds cause collagen damage.

3. Stop Skin Sabotage. I call them skin saboteurs, and they're all around us: foods that damage collagen. From refined carbs, to fried foods, to browned meats, a number of foods have been shown to accelerate the skin aging process.

EAT POWER

Eat power means eat foods that provide powerful nutrients. Certain foods contain the powerful nutrients that promote youthful skin. If you're looking at your dinner plate, you want to make sure you've got these covered.

- **Foods and beverages that are naturally rich in antioxidants,** including fruits, vegetables, green tea, herbs and spices, and more. These foods are also rich sources of anti-inflammatory compounds and other powerful nutrients, which means they pack a double punch.
- **Power carbs,** such as whole grains, beans, and lentils. These foods provide carbohydrates along with a host of powerful nutrients, including fiber, vitamins, minerals, phytonutrients, and protein.
- **Power fats,** including mono-unsaturated fatty acids (MUFAs) and omega-3 polyunsaturated fatty acids. These have been shown to help strengthen the skin barrier, maintain skin elasticity, and provide anti-inflammatory benefits.
- **Herbs and spices** are considered a triple threat: they're a concentrated, powerful source of antioxidants, they're a powerful source of anti-inflammatory compounds, and they have anti-glycation properties.
- **Prebiotics and probiotics** promote the growth of "good" microbes in the gastrointestinal (GI) tract. This ensures good gut health, and it impacts skin health. That's because these good gut microbes secrete substances that help strengthen the skin barrier and make it more resistant to irritation.

STOP SUGAR SPIKES

We all love cupcakes. But if you're enjoying them a little too frequently you're risking long-term collagen damage.

That's because eating foods heavy in refined carbohydrates or added sugars can cause elevated levels of blood sugar. That excess sugar can combine with proteins in the body to create advanced glycation end products (known as AGEs). These "sticky" compounds wreak havoc on your skin and on your health.

AGEs cause damage to collagen, blood vessels, and other organs. In the skin, that collagen damage results in sugar sag: premature wrinkling and sagging of the skin.

To prevent the formation of collagen-damaging AGEs, you need the right strategies. It starts by avoiding foods heavy in added sugars and refined carbs. It also means focusing on 3 main strategies:

- **Eat power carbs:** Carb sources such as whole grains, beans, and lentils naturally contain fiber. They also provide vitamins, minerals, phytonutrients, and sometimes protein.
- **The Half-Produce Plate:** With half your plate covered in fruits and vegetables, you're ensuring hefty doses of fiber and micronutrients.
- **Balanced Meals:** Eating meals that contain healthy protein to balance out carbs helps keep blood sugar levels stable.

STOP SKIN SABOTAGE

You may love doughnuts, but those deep-fried, sugary, carb-loaded treats are doing your skin no favors. They don't just cause your body to produce collagen-damaging AGEs. They actually contain their own pre-formed AGEs.

Your body produces AGEs when your blood sugar levels start to spike. But that's not the only way AGEs find their way into your collagen. You can also eat them. Pre-formed AGEs are found in browned meats, fried foods, some grilled foods, and others. Processed foods that contain trans fats are also skin saboteurs.

PUTTING IT ALL TOGETHER

Eat power. Stop sugar spikes. Stop skin sabotage.

When it comes to eating for youthful skin, these are the three major goals. And the right foods and recipes can help you reach them.

In the next chapter, you'll be introduced to some of the common (and less common) foods that promote youthful, luminous skin: skin saving foods.

CHAPTER 5
AN INTRODUCTION TO SKIN SAVING FOODS

Skin saving foods: from turmeric to broccoli to green tea, a number of foods have shown powerful skin benefits in research studies. In fact, research into the molecular mechanisms linking skin and nutrition has really exploded over the last few decades. As a result, there's been impressive progress into our understanding of how foods affect our skin. While more research needs to be done, these insights emphasize how important real foods are to health.

The following table highlights just some of the research and some of the foods and nutrients with powerful skin saving benefits. There are many, many more.

While I've listed single nutrients here, it's important to recognize that each food contains dozens and dozens of powerful nutrients. Some we've isolated and studied, and others are just waiting to be discovered. While you could list a dozen benefits for cauliflower alone, this table is meant to simply highlight some of the impressive benefits.

*While these foods have some great benefits, your medical profile will always determine what foods are great for you. Tomatoes, for example, protect against the damaging effects of UV radiation, but they can also trigger flares of rosacea in some individuals (chapter 23).

**Definitions and abbreviations are found at the end of the table

SKIN SAVING NUTRIENTS AND DERMATOLOGY RESEARCH

FOOD/ NUTRIENT	RESEARCH
VEGETABLES	
Artichokes/ Polyphenols	Potent antioxidant: per serving size, one of only 5 foods containing > 1000 mg of antioxidants per serving (out of 100 richest dietary sources)
Arugula/ Vitamin K	Necessary for blood clotting, important in wound healing
Asparagus/ Fiber	Very nutrient-dense: low in calories, but rich in vitamins, minerals, and prebiotic fiber
Avocado/ MUFAs	These power fats act to stabilize blood sugar levels following a meal
Beets/ Betalains	Pigments that provide the coloring of the beet as well as anti-inflammatory effects
Black beans/ Polyphenols	Per serving size, one of only 5 foods containing more than 1000 mg antioxidants per serving (out of 100 richest dietary sources evaluated)
Black olives/ Tyrosol	In one study, ranked as the richest vegetable source of polyphenols
Broccoli	Blocks DNA damage: After 10 days of eating broccoli every day, smokers experienced significantly less cellular DNA damage
Brussel sprouts	Blocks DNA damage: Volunteers eating Brussels sprouts every day experienced less DNA damage from oxidation
Cabbage/ Glucosinolates	Activates enzymes in liver that work to eliminate toxins from body

Carrots/ Beta-carotene	Potent antioxidant: strong skin protection demonstrated in many lab and animal studies
Cauliflower/ Quercetin	Protects collagen: acts to reduce the production of AGES
Celery/ Luteolin	Collagen protection: In the lab, this polyphenol was one of the strongest inhibitors of AGE production.
Chickpeas	Blood sugar control: In a study with human volunteers, long-term consumption of chickpeas improved blood sugar control
Corn/ Carotenoids	Good source of lutein and zeaxanthin, carotenoid antioxidants that in human studies protect against UV-induced skin damage
Cucumber	Low calorie, hydrating vegetable: flavonoids provide antioxidant benefits
Edamame/ Genistein	Antioxidant which scavenges pre-radicals and protects against cell membrane damage
Eggplant/ Phenolic acids	These phytonutrients are powerful free radical scavengers
Green beans/ Fiber	A nutrient-dense vegetable, with low calories and high fiber. In multiple studies, fiber has strong anti-inflammatory effects
Green lentils/ Protein, fiber, phytonutrients	Researchers evaluated volunteers' skin wrinkling using skin microscopy. The volunteers reporting a higher intake of legumes, fruits, vegetables, and extra-virgin olive oil had less skin wrinkling
Jicama/ Fiber	Serves as a prebiotic food by promoting the growth of good gut microbes: raw jicama sticks and dip are a simple snack
Kale/ Carotenoids	This leafy green vegetable provides a high concentration of antioxidant carotenoids, especially beta-carotene and lutein
Mushrooms/ Beta-glucans	This type of fiber has strong antioxidant properties in lab and animal studies

Onion/ Quercetin	Strong inhibitor of the collagen-destroying enzyme collagenase
Peas/ Fiber	Great source of anti-inflammatory and blood sugar-stabilizing fiber
Pepper, green/Luteolin	This phytonutrient inhibits the activity of collagenase, an enzyme that degrades collagen fibers
Pepper, orange/ Zeaxanthin	In a human experiment, ingestion of the carotenoids lutein and zeaxanthin reduced skin damage following UV radiation
Pepper, red/ Vitamin C	Quenches free radicals and regenerates vitamin E
Pumpkin/ Beta-cryptoxanthin	In laboratory studies, this carotenoid stimulates the repair of DNA damage
Red kidney beans/ Zinc	Zinc deficiency is more common in vegetarians, and can lead to skin inflammation by increasing levels of inflammatory chemical messengers
Red lentils/ Protein	Excellent source of plant-based protein
Romaine lettuce	This leafy green vegetable is known for its high nutrient density, with a very high NNR (naturally nutrient rich) score
Soybeans/ Genistein	Antioxidant which scavenges free radicals and protects against cell membrane damage
Spinach/ Iron	Adequate levels of iron are needed for hair growth
Squash, spaghetti/ Carotenoids	Low-calorie (only about 30 calories per cup), simple to cook, and a good source of carotenoid antioxidants

Sweet potatoes/ Beta carotene	Volunteers consuming more fruits and vegetables for 6 weeks had skin changes that were seen as more healthy, likely due to carotenoid pigments being incorporated into the skin.
Tomatoes/ Lycopene	In human subjects, 10 weeks of consumption led to decreased sunburn response and collagen damage
Zucchini/ Vitamin C	Considered a very nutrient-dense vegetable: with only 30 calories (approx.), one medium zucchini provides high levels of vitamin C and other vitamins and minerals

FRUITS

Apples/ Phloretin	This polyphenol is able to trap reactive molecules and thereby inhibit AGE formation
Apricots/ Carotenoids	Known for containing high levels and wide variety of carotenoids: after 4 weeks of eating fruits and veg high in carotenoids, volunteers had lower levels of systemic inflammation
Bananas/ Fiber	The fiber in this fruit serves as a prebiotic: it promotes the growth of good gut microbes
Berries/ Vitamin C	An essential cofactor in collagen biosynthesis
Blueberries/ Polyphenols	One of the richest food sources of these powerful phytonutrient antioxidants
Cantaloupe/ Vitamin C	A higher reported intake of vitamin C was associated with a lower likelihood of wrinkled skin and dryness
Cherries/ Anthocyanins	Potent antioxidants

Cranberries/ Vanillic acid	In lab studies, inhibits the collagen changes triggered by excess blood sugar
Dates/ Syringic acid	In lab studies, inhibits AGE production
Figs/ Rutin	In lab study, reduces collagen damage caused by AGEs
Fruit/ Gallic acid	Able to significantly block the glucose driven modification of proteins
Grapefruit/ Vanillic acid	In the laboratory, inhibits the protein changes triggered by excess blood sugar
Grapes/ Proanthocyanidins	In laboratory studies, these phytonutrients promote DNA repair
Kiwi/ Vitamin C	Higher intakes of vitamin C were associated with a lower likelihood of wrinkles and dry skin
Lemons/ Vitamin C	Potent antioxidant
Mangoes	In animal studies, consumption of a mango extract resulted in less skin aging following UV exposure
Oranges/ Flavonoids	In human volunteers, consuming citrus flavonoids and rosemary polyphenols/ diterpenes for 8 weeks resulted in enhanced skin protection against UV radiation
Peaches	DNA repair (following oxidative damage) was more efficient in animals fed a peach-enriched diet
Pears	A rich source of both fiber (approximately 5 g per pear) and polyphenol antioxidants

Pineapple/ Vitamin C	Quenches free radicals and regenerates vitamin E, another antioxidant
Plums/ Anthocyanins	These polyphenol phytonutrients provide plants with their blue/purple pigmentation, and have strong anti-inflammatory effects
Pomegranates/ Anthocyanins & Ellagic acid	Women who took pomegranate extract daily for four weeks experienced less skin damage from UV radiation
Raspberries/ Ellagic acid	In animal studies, consumption resulted in less redness and blistering after UV exposure
Starfruit	In laboratory studies, increased DNA repair in human skin cells after UV radiation
Strawberries/ Polyphenols	Known for their antioxidant abilities. In one lab study, a strawberry extract protected fibroblasts (important for collagen repair) from the damaging effects of free radicals
Watermelon/ Lycopene	This antioxidant reduces the skin damage that results from UV exposure

SPICES AND HERBS

Allspice	Inhibits production of collagen-damaging AGEs
Basil/ Apigenin	This flavonoid, in laboratory studies, was able to stimulate DNA repair genes after UV exposure
Cardamom	Dietary cardamom reduced skin cancer-like growths, likely via upregulation of detoxification enzymes, in an animal study
Cilantro/ Apigenin	May inhibit the collagen breakdown that occurs after exposure to UV radiation, as lab studies show that it inhibits the enzyme collagenase

Cinnamon	Some studies suggest that as little as 1/4 to 1/2 tsp daily reduces blood glucose levels, possibly by increasing the sensitivity of insulin receptors
Cloves	In one study, cloves had the highest antioxidant capacity (per 100 g) of all foods studied
Garlic/ Organosulfur compounds	Garlic reduced the formation of wrinkles following UVB exposure by protecting against collagen damage; compounds in garlic reduce oxidative stress and inflammation
Ginger/ Gingerols	Blocks activity of the enzyme elastase. This enzyme, triggered by UV radiation, acts to degrade elastic fibers
Mint	Strong antioxidant abilities
Nutmeg	In a lab study, nutmeg was found to block the "scissor" enzyme elastase.
Oregano/ Apigenin	This polyphenol compound scavenges ROS and inhibits the activity of collagenase, an enzyme that damages collagen
Paprika/ Beta-carotene	Potent antioxidant
Parsley/ Apigenin	Inhibitor of collagenase, an enzyme that degrades collagen
Peppermint/ Apigenin	In laboratory and animal studies, activated DNA repair systems and reduced inflammation after UV radiation
Rosemary/ Carnosol	This phytonutrient (terpene family) is a powerful antioxidant
Saffron	This spice has strong anti-inflammatory properties
Thyme/ Luteolin	In lab studies, protects fibroblasts (cells important in collagen repair) from UV radiation by scavenging free radicals
Turmeric/ Curcumin	Inhibits nuclear factor Kappa Beta, a major mediator of inflammation

GRAINS/NUTS/SEEDS

Almonds/ Vitamin E	Potent antioxidant: stabilizes cell membranes by preventing damage to fatty acids
Amaranth	This gluten-free grain of the Aztecs provides strong doses of both protein and fiber, in addition to minerals such as calcium, iron, and magnesium
Barley/ Beta glucan	This fiber helps control blood sugar
Brazil nuts/ Selenium	This antioxidant works with vitamin E to protect fatty acids in cell membranes from oxidation
Buckwheat/ Rutin	This gluten-free grain contains rutin, a phytonutrient which reduces collagen changes caused by AGEs
Bulgur/ Fiber	This whole grain food, made from whole wheat kernels, is a good source of fiber, important for gut health
Cashews/ Zinc	Adequate levels of zinc are important for hair growth
Chia seeds/ Fiber	Just 2 tablespoons of these seeds contain 5 g of protein and 10 g of fiber, which helps to stabilize blood sugar levels
Couscous, whole grain	Made from whole grain flour and easy to cook (cooking just requires soaking in boiling water)
Farro, whole	This ancient wheat contains high levels of protein and fiber
Flaxseed oil/ Omega-3s	After 12 weeks of daily consumption, subjects showed less water loss, less roughness, and less sensitivity of skin
Flaxseeds, freshly ground/ Omega-3s	Flaxseeds serve as a plant-based source of anti-inflammatory omega-3 fatty acids

Oats/ Beta-glucan fiber	Oats are a whole grain, with prebiotic fiber that encourages the growth of good microbes
Peanuts/ Niacin	The body uses niacin to produce nicotinamide, which has been shown to enhance DNA repair. In an experimental trial, volunteers given this nutrient for 1 year developed fewer skin cancers.
Pecans/ Manganese	Mineral needed for the normal functioning of different enzymes in the body, including one (prolidase) used in collagen production
Popcorn, home-cooked	Low-calorie, whole grain snack
Pistachios	Studies indicate that regular consumption of these nuts helps to stabilize blood sugar levels
Pumpkin seeds/ Zinc	Zinc deficiency is more common in vegetarians, and can lead to hair loss.
Quinoa/ 9 Essential amino acids	High in protein, fiber, and minerals, including manganese, magnesium, iron, and zinc
Rice, brown/ Selenium	This mineral is a potent antioxidant, with lab and animal studies supporting its role in skin cancer prevention
Sesame seeds/ Sesamin, a lignan	This polyphenol inhibits oxidative stress
Sunflower seeds/ Vitamin E and Selenium	Excellent source of these potent antioxidants: one of the top food sources of vitamin E
Walnuts/ Alpha linolenic acid, a type of omega-3 fatty acid	In one study, a higher reported intake of ALA from fruits, vegetables, and vegetable oils was associated with less photoaging

Whole wheat/ Ferulic acid	This polyphenol serves as an antioxidant and in lab studies acts to inhibit the glucose-triggered changes to proteins in the body
Wild rice/ Fiber	This seed of a grass has twice the protein and fiber of brown rice

OTHER

Apple Cider Vinegar/ Probiotics	Vinegars with "live" cultures of microbes are considered a probiotic food. Some of these "good" microbes have been demonstrated to reduce skin sensitivity and improve skin moisture.
Balsamic Vinegar/ Polyphenols	Since balsamic vinegar is made from grapes, it is a source of polyphenol antioxidants, which can combat the damaging effects of UV radiation
Broth, tamarind with spices (Indian rasam)	Combination of multiple anti-inflammatory and antioxidant herbs and spices
Coconut flour/ Fiber	High in fiber, with 5 grams of fiber per 2 tbsp. In one study, adding coconut flour to baked goods resulted in a lowering of glycemic index
Coffee/ Chlorogenic acids	In a study of Japanese women, higher reported intake of polyphenols from coffee and other sources was associated with a lower scoring of UV-related pigmented spots.
Dark chocolate/ Flavanols	After 12 weeks of consumption, high flavanol cocoa powder resulted in increased skin blood flow and hydration
Eggs/ Lutein	In a human experiment, ingestion of lutein with zeaxanthin, both carotenoids, reduced skin damage following UV radiation
Fermented milk/ Prebiotics and Probiotics	In a randomized experimental trial, consuming a fermented milk product that was rich in both prebiotics and probiotics acted to maintain skin hydration.

Kefir/ Multiple microbes	This fermented milk beverage is known for a high diversity of microbes, including numerous bacterial and yeast strains
Kimchi/	In human subjects, increased kimchi consumption for 7 days resulted in less pathogenic intestinal bacteria
Kombucha/ Probiotics	This fermented tea provides an easy to consume source of probiotics
Miso/ Probiotics	This fermented soy condiment is an easy-to-use source of good microbes; easily added to dips, sauces, and dressings
Olive oil	Higher reported intakes of olive oil were associated with less skin wrinkling
Peanut butter/ MUFAs	Good source of these healthy fats, in moderation
Salmon/ Omega-3s	Great source of anti-inflammatory long-chain omega-3 fatty acids
Sardines/ Vitamin D	May act to increase cathelicidin, a protein that has antimicrobial properties
Sauerkraut/ Probiotics	Certain types provide live, active cultures of beneficial bacteria
Scallops/ Protein	A low-calorie, high-protein seafood; also a great source of micronutrients, including vitamin B12 and the antioxidant selenium
Shrimp/ Protein	High protein content (building blocks for skin and hair) for a low calorie count
Tea, black	Drinking either black tea or green tea resulted in markedly lower numbers of skin cancer in animals exposed to UV radiation
Tea, chamomile/ Luteolin	Inhibits production of AGEs

Tea, green/ Polyphenols	In animal studies, these phytonutrient compounds aided in the repair of UVB-induced damage
Tea, matcha/ Catechins	This powdered green tea has a much higher concentration of the powerful antioxidant epigallocatechin gallate (EGCG) than even standard green tea
Tea, sencha/ EGCG	A Japanese green tea variety with high levels of epigallocatechin gallate (EGCG), a powerful antioxidant
Tea, white/	In one lab study, white tea was the strongest blocker of the skin-degrading enzymes collagenase and elastase
Tofu/ Isoflavones	Strong anti-inflammatory effects
Tuna/ Omega-3s	Strong anti-inflammatory properties
Vinegar	Consuming vinegar before a meal has been shown to reduce the sugar spikes that can occur after a carb-heavy meal.
Yogurt/ Lactobacillus and Bifidobacterium strains	Use in diabetic patients enhanced total antioxidant status, with increases in activity of superoxide dismutase and glutathione peroxidase

DEFINITIONS

Antioxidants	• Antioxidants are substances which are able to "quench" free radicals • This includes enzymes found within the body such as superoxide dismutase and glutathione peroxidase • Vitamins, minerals, and phytonutrients can also function as antioxidants • Some of the more well studied antioxidants include vitamin C, vitamin E, beta-carotene, and selenium
Flavonoids	• One of the major classes of polyphenols • Researchers have identified thousands of different flavonoids • These are divided into different categories based on chemical structure
Free Radicals	• Free radicals are molecules that contain unpaired electrons • They can cause direct damage to proteins, lipids, and DNA • Small amounts are generated from the body's everyday processes, with larger amounts generated from exposure to UV radiation and pollution
Glycation and AGEs	• Glycation occurs when a sugar molecule bonds with a protein or lipid • No enzyme is required for this bonding • This produces collagen-damaging compounds called advanced glycation end products (AGEs)

Phytonutrients	• These compounds are naturally found in plants • They provide plants with taste, color, smell, and other properties • Many protect plants from the sun, heat, insects, oxidative stress, and other threats • Three major categories include carotenoids, phenolic compounds, and organosulfur compounds
Polyphenols	• There are thousands of polyphenolic compounds • These are divided into different categories based on chemical structure • Different groups include flavonoids, stilbenes, tannins, phenolic acids, and lignans • Many plants contain polyphenols from different classes
Prebiotics and Probiotics	• Prebiotics promote the growth of "good" gut microbes • These microbes promote gut health and skin health • Most prebiotics are in the form of fiber from foods such as vegetables, legumes, and grains • Probiotics are foods or supplements that contain live, active cultures of good microbes
Reactive oxygen species (ROS)	• Most free radicals in the body exist in the form of reactive oxygen species

CHAPTER 6
THE SCIENCE OF AGING SKIN

While dermatologists have long known about the link between our diet and our skin, we now recognize that these are connected on a cellular level, in many different ways.

Is this new information?

No. We've actually known for centuries that our internal health and our skin health are closely related.

Take the skin changes seen in diabetes. One of the warning signs of diabetes is a darkening of the skin of the neck. This is known as acanthosis nigricans, and it indicates that the body isn't responding to insulin as well as it should (known as insulin resistance). When dermatologists diagnose acanthosis nigricans, we inform our patients that creams or even lasers are not the answer. This noticeable skin darkening is due to internal causes, and dietary changes are the key treatment.

It's also well-known that persons with diabetes have impaired wound healing. Their skin doesn't heal as well, due to changes in blood vessels and collagen. Those same changes can accelerate the skin aging process.

So, while the information isn't new, it's being studied much more intensively than ever before. Researchers have made great strides in uncovering the cellular mechanisms that link diet and the skin.

Why Does Our Skin Age?

When you're thinking about the link between your diet and your skin, it's helpful to start by thinking about the process of skin aging.

INTRINSIC AND EXTRINSIC FACTORS Some of the skin aging process has to do with what are known as intrinsic factors, such as the passage of time and our genetic makeup. Much of skin aging, though, is due to external factors. The one that most of us are familiar with is ultraviolet (UV) radiation from sun exposure. We've all seen actors on the big screen with this kind of skin aging – leathery, rough, deeply creased skin. Other external factors include pollution and (the very damaging) smoking.

PHYSICAL FORCES Physical forces can also impact our skin, and are a major force in aging skin: just think of smile lines and frown lines. Another major factor is gravity. Your skin eventually starts to sag and jowl in part because the collagen framework of your skin can no longer fight gravity as well.

When I started thinking about these factors, it made me wonder if there was any way to protect against these effects. Were there any foods that could protect against the damaging effects of UV radiation? Was there any way to strengthen the collagen so that it could better withstand the forces of gravity?

It turns out that yes, dietary changes can actually protect you from some of the forces that accelerate aging of the skin.

Your Skin Is Under Siege

You don't necessarily think about it every day, but your skin stands guard to protect you from multiple threats. From the elements, to extremes of temperature, to staph bacteria, your skin stands guard every day.

You can think of your skin as a house. Just like a house, your skin provides shelter and protection.

And you need that protection, because the threats to your skin come at you from all sides. Here are the big three, which I think of as **OMG**:

- ♦ **OXIDATIVE STRESS** due to UV radiation and pollution causing free radicals
- ♦ **MAJOR AND MINOR INFLAMMATION** due to your body's defense and repair processes going haywire in response to signals
- ♦ **GLYCATION** due to excess blood sugar

The right foods can combat each of these forces.

Oxidative Stress: Free Radicals Pounding The Skin

You need to make sure that your skin stands guard against UV radiation. Just like rain and hail can pound the roof of your home, the free radicals that are formed from UV radiation and pollution can pummel your skin and damage DNA, skin proteins (such as collagen and elastic fibers), and lipids (such as cell membranes). To quench those free radicals, you need antioxidants, especially the kind found in certain foods.

Inflammation: Defense And Repair Processes Out Of Control

You also need to make sure that your body's repair processes work exactly as designed. Just like an overzealous repairman who starts by fixing one small leak but ends by creating a large hole in your roof, your repair processes can sometimes result in more damage than repair. That's chronic inflammation: when the body's repair processes start to go haywire. An anti-inflammatory diet can act to calm down the process of inflammation.

Glycation: The Creation Of "Sticky", Damaging Compounds That Weaken The Skin's Structure

You also need to worry about the collagen fibers that form the structural basis of your skin. Just like termites can eat away at the walls of your home, advanced glycation end products, which are formed from excess sugar in your system, can weaken the collagen framework that supports your skin. To combat glycation, you need to focus on the right foods to keep blood sugar levels stable.

Other Threats

I think of these as the three major threats to your skin health, but they're certainly not the only ones.

Hormones have many potential effects on your skin, and some changes in hormone levels can stress and damage your skin. Just like extremes of temperature can warp the walls of your home, changes in hormone levels can change the functioning of the skin barrier, the strength of the collagen framework, and other skin properties. These include hormones such as thyroid hormone, estrogen, and the stress hormone cortisol.

It's All Connected

As in so much of medicine, skin aging is due to a combination of these factors and others, and they're all interrelated. Exposure to UV exposure can cause free radical production. Those free radicals can cause direct damage to collagen and DNA. They can also activate the body's defense and repair systems, leading to more damage from inflammation. The process of glycation weakens the collagen framework, and that weakening is accelerated in areas already stressed by oxidation.

How Exactly Do Foods Combat Skin Aging?

The right foods can combat each of these processes, whether that's via antioxidants, anti-inflammatory nutrients, anti-glycation properties, or other effects. The next section describes these foods and the research behind them.

CHAPTER 7
THE SCIENCE BEHIND SKIN SAVING NUTRIENTS: EAT POWER

Eat power means focus on **eating foods that are rich in powerful nutrients**.

These 6 categories of foods have been shown to help the skin.

- **Foods that are naturally rich in antioxidants:** This includes foods such as herbs and spices, fruits and vegetables, and green tea. These foods are also anti-inflammatory, so they provide a double dose of beneficial effects.

- **Power carbs:** Foods such as whole grains, beans, and lentils contain carbohydrates combined in a package with antioxidants, fiber, and protein.

- **Power fats:** These include certain MUFAs and PUFAs.

- **Herbs and spices:** Multiple herbs and spices have been shown to protect collagen by fighting the processes of oxidation, inflammation, and glycation.

- **Probiotic foods:** These foods contain live, active cultures of "good" microbes.

- **Prebiotic foods:** These foods naturally promote the growth of good bacteria in your gut. The fiber found in many vegetables can be a powerful prebiotic.

How Do These Powerful Nutrients Work to Help the Skin?

◆ Dietary antioxidants combat the cellular damage inflicted by UV radiation.

Certain foods can combat the damage inflicted by UV radiation. This damage is known as photoaging. We know that chronic sun exposure, over years, changes the skin in fundamental ways. **The damage inflicted by UV radiation can ultimately lead to fine lines and wrinkles, freckling and sun spots, loss of elasticity, and thinning of the skin**.

Research has shown that certain antioxidants in food can actually prevent, on a cellular level, some of the damage inflicted by UV radiation. For example, tomato paste eaten before exposure to UV radiation actually limited the sunburn response. This isn't the same as sunscreen, of course, but it adds an extra level of protection against the damaging effects of the sun's rays.

In one study, subjects who ate close to 2 tablespoons of tomato paste daily for 10 weeks showed less of a sunburn response after UV exposure.

Researchers have studied a number of antioxidants found in foods. In laboratory studies, animal studies, and even some human studies, these antioxidants have shown significant promise. They're able to block, and sometimes even repair, some of the cellular damage caused by UV radiation. Some antioxidants neutralize reactive oxygen species [which cause skin damage]. Some block the action of "scissor enzymes" such as collagenase and elastase, which damage the collagen and elastic fibers that provide strength and resiliency to your skin. Some foods are even able to mobilize the body's own DNA repair systems.

Antioxidants demonstrating skin-protective effects in research studies

♦ **RESVERATROL** in red grapes
♦ **LYCOPENE** in tomatoes and tomato paste
♦ **ELLAGIC ACID** in raspberries
♦ **CATECHINS** in green tea
♦ **CURCUMIN** in turmeric

This is just a sample of the powerful antioxidants found in foods: there appear to be thousands more in fruits, vegetables, spices, herbs, seeds, and nuts.

Why do I emphasize eating these foods instead of just taking an antioxidant pill? Because the studies that have tested supplements with isolated antioxidants have shown that they just don't work the same way as the antioxidants supplied in foods.

Researchers aren't sure exactly why this is, but I believe it's because whole foods provide fiber and many other phytonutrients, and the synergy of these substances promotes their beneficial effects. [Synergy means that substances acting together are more powerful than those substances acting alone. This has been demonstrated in multiple laboratory studies.]

◆ **Eating "power" carbs instead of refined carbs has several powerful skin benefits.**

Why do I consider lentils, beans, sweet potatoes, and whole grains to be power carbs? It's because these foods are a great source of several powerful nutrients.

Consuming power carbs in place of refined carbs [meaning more whole grains and lentils and less white bread and white rice], can help your skin in several ways.

◆ **Powerful Source of Antioxidants:** Beans, as one example, provide selenium, a mineral that's been shown to help fight oxidation. In laboratory and animal studies, selenium has even helped to reduce the incidence of skin cancer. That's only one nutrient. There are many, many other phytonutrients found in beans, lentils, whole grains, and vegetables. Researchers have only just started to uncover their many benefits.

◆ **Hefty Dose of Prebiotic Fiber:** Fiber is considered an incredibly important nutrient, even though we don't always hear that message. We hear celebrities talk about eating more protein, and we've all been told to make sure we're getting enough vitamins and minerals. The message of "eat more fiber" isn't as popular, but it's incredibly important for our health and our skin. [When I say fiber, I mean real, food-based fiber, like the type you find in beans and vegetables. The highly processed fiber that's added to protein bars and protein shakes hasn't yet been shown to function in the body in the same way as real fiber, so I'm leery of relying on fake fiber for health benefits.]

Researchers are still discovering the amazing properties of fiber. To start with, the fiber found in certain vegetables, beans, lentils, and whole grains functions as a powerful prebiotic. Prebiotics are substances that act to promote the growth of "good microbes" in our gut. Those good microbes have been shown to help strengthen your skin barrier and tame inflammation.

◆ **Hefty dose of Fiber and Extra Dose of Protein to Stabilize Blood Sugar Levels:** The carbohydrates in beans, lentils, and whole grains come packaged with a hefty dose of fiber and protein. Fiber and protein act to stabilize blood sugar levels, which in turn helps preserve collagen.

◆ Eating "power" fats may help your skin barrier function.

The first time I read about this, I thought it sounded a little too good to be true. Could eating more fat actually "moisturize" your skin from the inside? It turns out that this is true. The right kind and the right levels of fat in your diet (not too little and definitely not too much) can help optimize the function

Volunteers who consumed flaxseed oil daily for 12 weeks showed less skin irritation after exposure to an irritating substance. They also retained moisture better.

of your skin barrier. This has been demonstrated for certain monounsaturated fatty acids (MUFAs) and for omega-3 polyunsaturated fatty acids (PUFAs). These "good" fats also have anti-inflammatory properties, which helps to limit skin damage.

A few examples of foods that supply fats (along with other powerful nutrients):

- **Nuts:** walnuts, Brazil nuts, almonds, pecans
- **Seeds:** chia seeds, ground flaxseeds
- **Vegetables:** avocados, olives, olive oil
- **Fatty fish:** herring, mackerel, salmon, sardines, trout, tuna

◆ Herbs and Spices: A Skin-Saving Triple Threat

Herbs and spices are what I call a triple threat. They combat oxidation AND inflammation AND glycation, which are the three major forces that age your skin.

Herbs and spices provide a potent, concentrated source of antioxidants. In fact, research studies looking at the antioxidant capacity of multiple foods consistently rank herbs and spices at the top. These same herbs and spices also have potent anti-inflammatory properties.

Herbs and spices also battle glycation. Glycation occurs in the presence of higher blood sugars and results in the formation of advanced glycation end products (AGEs). These "sticky" compounds cause collagen damage. Some spices help prevent the formation of AGEs, while others limit the collagen damage that results. Some may even help reduce blood sugar levels in the first place.

◆ Prebiotic and probiotic foods help the skin barrier.

It may sound far-fetched, but research has found that the microbes that live in your gut have the ability to help your skin. We call this the gut-skin connection.

There are many microbes that live in your gastrointestinal (GI) tract, and these microbes have the ability to affect many of your body's functions. This includes the function of your immune system, your metabolism, and your skin barrier. Studies have found that more "good" microbes in your GI tract may result in a more effective skin barrier. This translates to less moisture loss from the skin, along with less sensitivity to irritation.

How can you ensure that your gut contains these good microbes? You need to start by feeding them the right food. And that means fiber. The fiber found in certain foods acts as a "prebiotic", which means that it helps encourage the growth of good microbes.

In some cases, you may also be able to consume these good microbes. "Probiotics" refers to foods or supplements that contain live active cultures of good microbes. Several studies have demonstrated an improvement in skin barrier function with probiotics.

> In research studies, the consumption of synbiotics (which are combinations of probiotics with prebiotics) has improved the skin of some patients with eczema.

CHAPTER 8
THE SCIENCE BEHIND GLYCATION

Fine lines and wrinkles. A deepening of smile lines. A softening of the jawline. These are common signs of aging skin, and they reflect collagen damage. And one of the major threats to your collagen is sugar. Specifically, excess sugar in your bloodstream.

Excess sugar can combine with proteins in your body and create collagen-damaging molecules. That's why one of the keys to eating for younger skin is "stop sugar spikes."

Collagen Is Strong, Flexible, And Extremely Resilient

Collagen is one of the major skin proteins, and it's what makes our skin so strong and at the same time so flexible and resilient. Your skin is an amazing organ, especially when you think about all of the functions that it has to perform. It maintains a protective skin barrier, and it helps our skin move with us and then bounce right back. The collagen fibers in your skin are able to accomplish that, partly because of the fact that they're arrayed in the skin so well. I think of collagen fibers as similar to a net: closely and carefully arrayed, so that they can be strong yet flexible.

That strong flexible foundation, though, can be damaged. Ultraviolet radiation is one of the biggest threats to your collagen. Sun exposure, over time, causes cumulative damage to collagen on a microscopic level. But UV radiation isn't the only threat to your collagen. Sugar is another.

Higher Blood Glucose Levels Threaten Collagen

When you experience higher levels of sugar in your bloodstream (known as blood glucose), some of that sugar attaches to proteins. In a process known as glycation, excess sugar attaches to proteins and creates new molecules known as AGEs (advanced glycation end products).

AGEs Are Sugar-Protein Molecules That Act Like Caramel Tangling Up A Collagen Net

I think of AGEs as similar to caramel. If you combine sugar and butter, you end up with gooey, sticky, golden caramel. As that caramel hardens, it becomes hard and brittle. AGEs, just like caramel, are sticky: they act to cross-link your collagen fibers. That ultimately leads to wrinkling and sagging of your skin.

Think of what would happen if you added caramel to a net: you'd end up with a tangled mess that wouldn't function very well. It's the same with your collagen fibers, with the effect being a loss of resiliency. To make things worse, your collagen, once it's been cross-linked by AGEs, becomes more brittle and harder to repair. That "harder to repair" part is important, because it accelerates the aging process. As your skin loses its resiliency, you'll start to see more wrinkling and sagging.

Sugar Sag Is Irreversible, But It Is Preventable

This process is known as sugar sag, and it's irreversible. Once your collagen becomes cross-linked, there's no way to undo that process.

That's why it's so important to focus on prevention. And it's the reason "stop sugar spikes" is one of my key tenets of eating for healthy skin: it's important to keep your blood sugar levels stable so that they can't contribute to making more AGEs.

AGEs Impact Many Organ Systems

Eating for skin health means eating for health. AGEs don't just impact the collagen in your skin. They impact many other organs, such as your blood vessels. That's important, because once your blood vessels lose their flexibility, they put you at higher risk for diseases such as hypertension and heart disease.

To Protect Your Collagen, Protect Against Sugar Spikes

This is one of the reasons why that bedtime bowl of ice cream isn't the best choice. Foods with added sugars, or foods that contain refined carbohydrates, or even too large a serving of whole grains, can all lead to rapid increases in your blood sugar levels. These are known as "sugar spikes", and they're problematic. If you want to protect your collagen, it's important to limit those sugar spikes.

> In one study, strictly controlling blood sugar levels over a 4-month period resulted in a 25% reduction of glycated collagen formation.

Chapter 18 goes over the tweaks that you can make that limit these damaging elevations in blood sugar. Surprisingly, some foods actually contain high levels of pre-formed AGEs; the next chapter discusses these foods.

CHAPTER 9
STOP SKIN SABOTAGE

It's Friday afternoon, and you're finally headed out of town. You've been looking forward to this road trip for weeks. As dinnertime hits and you pull off the highway, you can almost taste your classic road trip meal. A broiled all-beef hamburger patty on a soft white bread bun. A side of beautiful golden crisp French fries. A tall plastic cup filled to the brim with fizzy carbonated cola. And your childhood favorite: a deep-fried apple pie to finish it off.

A classic road trip meal. And a great recipe for skin sabotage.

This meal is full of what I call "skin saboteurs": the foods and ingredients that act to pound away at your collagen from the inside.

- **Added sugars and refined carbs:** Sugar-loaded beverages, sugar-loaded desserts, and carb-loaded buns and potatoes all ramp up your blood sugar levels, which ramps up your production of AGEs.
- **Foods loaded with AGEs:** Certain foods are loaded with pre-formed skin-damaging AGEs. This especially includes browned meats (including broiled, grilled, and pan-fried), and all types of fried foods.
- **Foods heavy in trans fats:** Processed foods made with partially hydrogenated oils, and foods fried in these oils, trigger free radical formation in the skin.

All of which adds up to a meal that's a recipe for skin sabotage.

AGEs Are A Threat To Collagen

In the preceding section, you learned about the danger of advanced glycation end products (AGEs). There are two kinds of AGEs:

- The kind that you make in your body
- The kind that you eat in your food

•The kind you make in your body: Your body forms these sugar-protein compounds in response to excess blood sugar in your system. If you think of the collagen fibers that support your skin as a strong, flexible net, then AGEs are the caramel that tangle that net.

•The kind that you eat in your food: While your body can create AGEs, you can also eat them. We call these pre-formed AGEs, and certain foods are loaded with them. This includes meat and some processed foods.

How you cook your food matters also. Certain cooking methods greatly increase the formation of AGEs, especially the cooking methods that create nice brown crusts: grilling at high temperatures, broiling, pan-frying, and deep-frying. One of the highest levels of AGEs are found in (wait for it) that sizzling crisp strip of bacon. Other top sources are foods such as whipped butter that have been subjected to certain processing methods.

Trans Fats Also Age Your Skin

If there's one thing everybody agrees on, it's that you shouldn't be consuming trans fats. These chemicals were produced in a laboratory to help food last for years on a shelf While they're a known danger to overall health, they also present a danger to the skin: research has shown that they increase the production of collagen-damaging free radicals.

Thankfully, the use of trans fats and partially hydrogenated vegetable oils (which lead to the formation of more trans fats) will be banned in the United States starting in 2018. While trans fats can be found in small amounts in some natural foods, such as beef, cheese, and full-fat dairy, they're mainly found in processed shelf-stable foods (cookies and crackers) or foods fried in partially hydrogenated vegetable oils (such as some restaurant French fries).

CHAPTER 10
PUTTING IT INTO PRACTICE

While the preceding chapters have focused on the cellular mechanisms behind the dietary recommendations, the next chapters focus on action. In section 2, you'll learn more about skin-saving foods. In section 4, you'll find recipes that incorporate these foods.

A few key points on eating for healthy skin:

- **The right foods**: The right foods are more important than any one nutrient.
- **The right meals:** Your overall pattern of eating is more important than any individual food.
- **The right foods for you:** Everybody has a unique biochemical profile, which means your response to a food may be different than someone else's.

The recommendations throughout this book focus on an overall eating pattern that emphasizes whole foods over processed foods. It's an eating pattern that emphasizes whole foods as opposed to specific nutrients or supplements. It relies on a hefty dose of vegetables, along with a variety of foods that contain powerful nutrients.

This is the type of dietary pattern that's supported by the research behind the Mediterranean diet, the DASH diet, and the MIND diet. And it's the same type of diet we recommend to promote skin health.

Laws Of Food

A few important points about the science behind diet and dermatology and how this translates to the real world:

- Certain nutrients are important for skin health.
- But foods are far more powerful than nutrients. A single head of cauliflower combines dozens of nutrients.
- A meal is more important than a single food, because eating patterns (the combination of foods that you eat) are more powerful than any single food.

A single head of cauliflower combines dozens of nutrients: some we know about, and others are still waiting to be discovered. These dozens of nutrients may each have a separate, important health benefit. That's why just taking a capsule of quercetin isn't going to replicate the benefits of cauliflower.

CAULIFLOWER: A SKIN SAVING FOOD

Fiber	Prebiotic: enhances the growth of good gut microbes
Vitamin C	A powerful antioxidant and essential for collagen biosynthesis
Vitamin K	Used in the process of blood clotting
Folate	Used in cell repair
Glucosinolates	Phytonutrient compounds; detoxify harmful substances
Quercetin	Quenches free radicals
Rutin	Inhibits production of AGEs

Overall Eating Patterns Are More Important Than Any Single Nutrient Or Food

Foods are more powerful than nutrients. And your overall eating pattern-what you eat in the course of an entire week-is more important than any one food. This next recipe demonstrates this principle, because just this one snack packs in a whole host of skin-saving nutrients.

Skin Saving Snacks: Roasted Cauliflower With Romesco Sauce

Roasted cauliflower with Romesco sauce is a simple recipe: just bake the cauliflower, and just blend the ingredients for the sauce. Here's what you get from this simple recipe:

- Cauliflower is a great source of the flavonoid compound quercetin, a potent antioxidant.
- Red peppers are a great source of vitamin C, a powerful antioxidant and a vitamin essential for collagen biosynthesis.
- Almonds are very high in vitamin E, an important defender against free radicals.
- Garlic contains phytonutrients called organosulfur compounds, which have powerful anti-inflammatory effects.
- Paprika provides a concentrated source of beta-carotene, another skin-protecting antioxidant.
- Olive oil provides monounsaturated fatty acids (MUFAs), which help in the maintenance of a well-functioning skin barrier. They also improve your body's absorption of carotenoids (which includes beta-carotene.)

But even that list of impressive benefits doesn't even begin to cover what you get. Here's a longer list of the nutrients found in this skin-saving snack:

INGREDIENT	SKIN-SAVING NUTRIENTS
CAULIFLOWER	Vitamin C, Quercetin, Fiber, Vitamin K, Folate, Glucosinolates
RED PEPPERS	Vitamin C, Beta-carotene, Lutein, Vitamin B6, Fiber
ALMONDS	Vitamin E, MUFAs, Calcium, Potassium, Fiber
GARLIC	Organosulfur compounds
PAPRIKA	Beta-Carotene, Lutein, Vitamin B6, Vitamin E
OLIVE OIL	MUFAs (aid in absorption of carotenoids), Polyphenols

CHAPTER 11
THE LAWS OF MEDICINE AND NUTRITION

As a dermatologist, I know how challenging and frustrating skin concerns can be. While researchers continue to seek out safe, effective answers, we still have a long way to go to unravel the intricacies of the human body. Here are just a few of the different factors that physicians consider when evaluating research studies and developing health recommendations.

Laws Of Medicine

- First, do no harm.
- Everybody is unique, with a unique genetic profile and biochemical profile.
- Your body changes over time.
- The human body is amazing and mysterious.

First, Do No Harm.

The science of skin care has made some truly amazing leaps in the last few decades, with advances in sun protection, skin care, dermatology procedures, and laser technologies. However, my area of expertise is in allergic reactions of the skin, which means I'm very, very cautious about new products and procedures. If you're thinking about using/ getting one of these, always seek experienced, knowledgeable advice.

> **For new treatments, always apply the ASE test.**
>
> Is this product or pill or procedure or strategy:
>
> - Affordable
> - Safe
> - And Effective?
>
> A diet based on nutrient-rich, power-packed foods passes this test.

That's one of the reasons I'm so passionate about promoting dietary changes to maintain younger skin and promote overall health: they're safe and effective. And dietary changes can also be an important addition in the treatment of some skin conditions, such as acne and rosacea.

On the other hand, not all dietary changes are safe. Extremely restrictive diets, high fat diets, high protein diets, high carb diets: all of them can result in real medical consequences, and need to be approached with care and caution.

Everybody Is Different: The Need For Personalized Medicine

What's the first thing you do when you get to your doctor's office? You sit down and fill out those long medical history forms.

That's because we're all different. And those differences have a strong impact on how we react to different foods and nutrients. While multiple studies have proven this fact, we need a lot more research to untangle all of the different factors that impact our response to food.

◆ **Genetics** Why is it that some people can lose 20 pounds on a particular diet, while others gain 10 pounds on the same exact plan? If you look at the many weight loss experimental trials that have been published, there's always a wide variability in how individuals respond to the same exact diet.

Some of this may be due to genetics.

> Can you lose weight on a high-protein diet? You can if you have the right genes.
>
> Researchers put volunteers on a high-protein diet, and then measured how much weight they lost. Those who had a particular genetic marker lost significantly more weight on the high-protein diet.

Another study looked at low-fat diets and a different genetic marker. Patients with this genetic marker did better on the low-fat diet (than those without the marker). These patients had more weight loss and showed greater improvements in blood glucose and insulin levels on a low-fat diet.

There's a whole lot more fascinating research on this subject. One excellent summary article (listed in the references at the end of the book), by Dr. Lu Qi, is titled "Gene-Diet Interactions and Weight Loss."

◆ **Gut microbiome** You might expect that every volunteer in a medical study who's asked to follow a lower calorie, higher fiber diet would go on to lose weight. (That sounds like a great weight loss plan.) However, the composition of their gut microbiome (meaning the types of microbes that lived in their GI tract) actually impacted how much weight these volunteers lost. Volunteers with a particular type of bacteria (*Akkermansia muciniphila*) in their gut lost more weight.

◆ **Medications** It's well-known that certain medications can lead to weight gain, such as steroids and certain antidepressants. Even antibiotics are under suspicion.

> Researchers went looking for a way to help chickens pack on the pounds. They found it: antibiotics.
>
> Chickens who were given antibiotics grew faster and bigger.

Research is ongoing into whether eating these antibiotic-treated chickens would impact your own tendency to gain weight. There's also research looking into whether antibiotic use in people would have the same effects.

◆ **Medical History** Your medical history also affects your responses to nutrients. For example, women with polycystic ovarian syndrome may be more sensitive to carbohydrates.

◆ **Other Factors** Some people can eat a banana, and their blood sugar barely budges. Another person may see their blood sugar levels shoot up after eating that same banana. We don't yet understand all of the factors that decide how your body is going to respond to different nutrients. One study demonstrated these individual differences well.

> Researchers asked 800 volunteers to wear a continuous glucose monitoring device and then measured their blood sugar levels. They found startling differences.
>
> After eating the same exact meal, some people had very high blood sugar levels (sugar spikes) while others had blood sugar levels that barely budged.

Why would there be such dramatic differences? When looking at the possible explanations for these different blood sugar responses to the same exact meals, researchers found associations with weight, age, C-reactive protein levels (a measure of inflammation in the body), blood pressure, and even the composition of the gut bacteria.

Your body changes over time.

While you may not look the same as you did years ago, the changes in your body go far deeper than just appearance alone. Many of the body's systems and hormones change with age. For example, you may not be able to process carbohydrates as well.

One research study found that in older women (as compared to younger women), their blood sugar and insulin levels stayed elevated longer after a large meal. That may be one reason why you could easily handle a giant bowl of breakfast cereal as a teenager, but just can't anymore.

The human body is amazing and mysterious.

As much as we've researched and studied and learned, the human body remains amazing and mysterious.

The best scientists all emphasize one important point: we don't yet have all the answers, and we need to support well-designed, well-conducted, and strongly funded research.

When it comes to diet and skin care questions, sometimes these rules come into play. They may sound obvious, but they're not necessarily obvious when you're the one impacted by skin changes. Here are a few of the common inquiries I've heard from patients:

———————————

"Why would I have dry skin now? I never did before."

Your body changes with time, and so does your skin. In fact, as we age, our skin tends to lose its ability to retain moisture.

———————————

"This book says dairy is bad for you. Should I give it up?"

In response, I always ask: Who are you? And what do you mean by dairy?

Who are you? One of the laws of medicine: everybody is different. When it comes to dairy, infants and children grow and thrive well with cow's milk (dairy is good for them) and we don't recommend elimination unless there's a reason. On the other hand, there are some people with eczema (not all) whose dairy allergy makes their skin flare, and some people with acne (not all) whose skin worsens when they consume dairy (dairy is not good for them).

And what do you mean by dairy? Are you talking about 24 ounces a day of skim milk from corn-fed cows treated with antibiotics and hormones, or are you talking about one daily serving of organic fermented dairy (yogurt)? Researchers are still trying to untangle all the nuances of these different versions of dairy.

———————————

"I have no family history of psoriasis. Why do I have psoriasis?"

This is one of the biggest questions in dermatology, and despite all of our research, we still don't know for sure. Genetic factors, environmental factors, inflammatory factors, hormonal factors: the cause is likely due to the interplay of many factors, and we definitely need more research.

This last question emphasizes one point: there are still many areas within medicine, and definitely within nutrition, where we don't yet know the answer. The human body is a miracle and a mystery, and it's one of the reasons more research into chronic skin diseases is so necessary.

In the area of diet and dermatology, research has really exploded over the last 1-2 decades. I would not have been able to write this book at the start of my career, because much of the research hadn't been done yet. Through the efforts of many dedicated scientists and clinicians, the link between our skin and our diet continues to be explored and charted. There are still many unanswered questions, and in some sections of the book I've indicated that more research is needed. In others, I rely on the combined results of multiple studies that support certain recommendations. I keep a close eye on scientific developments in this area, and I highlight some of these on my blog (SkinAndDiet.com).

Laws Of Nutrition

- There is an optimal level of almost every nutrient. Too little, and you're at risk for deficiency. Too much, and you're at risk for toxicity.
- Nutrients working together in harmony are more powerful than any single nutrient.
- The human body is a finely balanced system, and so are the body's processes, such as oxidation.

The Goldilocks Principle: There is an optimal "just right" level for every nutrient.

It's just like Goldilocks and her porridge-not too hot, and not too cold, but just right. In the case of nutrients, you're looking for not too little (deficiency) and not too much (toxicity), but just right (optimal).

Take vitamin A. Vitamin A is critical to good health. In fact, vitamin A deficiency is a leading cause worldwide of blindness. If you consume too much though (usually via high-dose supplements), vitamin A is dangerous. We even have a name for the ingestion of high doses: hypervitaminosis A. In this condition, patients experience dry skin, dry eyes, hair loss, and even liver damage.

This is one of the reasons I'm so concerned about the lack of regulation and the indiscriminate use of supplements. Take hair loss. If your hair loss supplement contains vitamin A, and you're taking a multivitamin that also contains it, you may start to develop levels that are too high. That, ironically, can actually worsen hair loss.

When you're consuming nutrients through a combination of foods (a balanced diet) you're more likely to reach those optimal levels. Supplements may be useful in some cases, but they have to be chosen carefully: the right supplement at the right dose for the right condition.

The Symphony Principle: Instruments playing together, in harmony, make beautiful music.

Think of the beautiful clear sound of a flute. Now slowly add in all of the other instruments in a symphony. The music has changed: it's now more complex and more powerful and more stirring.

It's the same with nutrients. In medicine, we call this synergy, and it's been demonstrated many times. Nutrients acting together produce far more powerful health benefits than you would expect by just adding together their individual effects. In dermatology research, using four powerful antioxidants together produced far greater results than just one antioxidant alone.

This is one of the reasons experts emphasize foods over supplements. Foods are considered "nature's perfect package." A single carrot combines vitamins, minerals, phytonutrients, and fiber. And that combination has powerful health benefits. It's also one of the reasons we emphasize overall eating patterns more than any one food.

Hummus with carrot sticks is a powerful skin-saving recipe, because the vitamins, minerals, fiber, and phytonutrients in chickpeas, carrots, sesame seeds, olive oil, paprika, and garlic all multiply each other's benefits.

The Marching Band Principle: If the drums get too loud, it all sounds off.

All of the instruments in a marching band playing together make powerful, stirring music. If just one of those instruments is off, though, it's very jarring. It's the same with many of the body's systems. The human body is an amazing, carefully balanced system. If you take one hormone (such as thyroid hormone) and send it too high or too low, your body starts to compensate. This sets off a cascade of effects, some of which you experience as painful symptoms.

The same is true of nutrients. The antioxidants in foods are powerful health-promoting nutrients, but the whole process of oxidation and anti-oxidation is a finely balanced system. Supplements of isolated antioxidants just don't function in the body the way that antioxidants in foods function.

Research study after research study has found that supplements such as vitamin E and beta-carotene, which are so amazing in the lab, just aren't as beneficial when you take them as single supplements (as opposed to in foods).

> One study found that smokers taking beta-carotene supplements actually had <u>higher</u> rates of lung cancer.

This is one of the reasons I'm so focused on whole foods and recipes that incorporate whole foods: consuming a diet rich in a variety of whole foods means that you're able to benefit from synergy AND that you're able to naturally consume nutrients such as antioxidants in the right balance.

GLOW

Section 2

WHAT TO EAT

CHAPTER 12
ANTIOXIDANTS

- ◆ What are antioxidants?
- ◆ Why are they so important for healthy skin?
- ◆ How can I consume more?

Antioxidants in the body combat the skin damage caused by free radicals. They're constantly being depleted, which means the antioxidants supplied by the foods you eat are an important source of renewed protection.

A study on common foods in the US diet found that spices, herbs, nuts, seeds, berries, fruits, and vegetables contained the highest levels of antioxidants.

Your Skin Is Under Siege By Free Radicals

Your skin is under siege. Every minute of every day. Just living and breathing results in the production of molecules in the body called free radicals. These molecules contain an unpaired electron, which makes them unstable and potentially damaging. In fact, these molecules can damage your skin's proteins, lipids, and DNA. That means an acceleration of the aging process, and even an increase in the risk of skin cancer. Your body, though, is prepared for this onslaught.

Your Skin Contains Antioxidants, Which Stand Ready To Quench Free Radicals

Your skin contains many antioxidants, especially in the outermost layer of the skin (the epidermis). We call these "innate" skin antioxidants, and they include enzymes such as superoxide dismutase and glutathione peroxidase. Your skin also contains other antioxidants, including vitamin C, vitamin E, and beta carotene.

These antioxidants stand ready to quench free radicals. They do this by donating an electron, which stabilizes the free radical.

Sometimes Your Skin's Protective Systems Are Overwhelmed

Exposure to UV radiation and pollution generates free radicals, sometimes too many for the system to handle. When this happens, you start to see skin damage.

After sun exposure, you may see some skin damage immediately, such as the redness of a sunburn. But most of the damage from daily UV exposure takes place on a cellular level, with DNA damage and collagen breakdown.

Over time, that cellular damage produces visible damage. That's when you'll start to see fine lines and wrinkles, a loss of elasticity, and a noticeable increase in dark spots.

These are the outward signs of years of cellular skin damage.

Free radicals also damage the skin in another way: they incite inflammation. When certain proteins in your skin are damaged by free radicals, they send out signals that activate inflammation. That inflammation can then lead to even more skin damage.

The Antioxidants In Your Foods Are An Important Source Of Renewable Skin Protection

The antioxidants found in your diet can prevent this damage. In fact, it's important to keep renewing your skin's supply of antioxidants via foods, since they're constantly being used up in the process of battling free radicals.

Luckily, the foods in your diet can replenish your skin's store of antioxidants. The right foods have been shown to reduce the damage caused by UV radiation. Finding ways to incorporate these foods into every meal can provide for ongoing, renewable skin protection.

> One study looked at the antioxidant content of over 1100 food products commonly consumed in the United States (based on consumption data).
>
> Only 87 foods contained a significant amount of antioxidant content per serving size.

Antioxidants in Your Diet: Vitamins, Minerals, Phytonutrients, and More

Antioxidants are defined by their function, not by their chemical structure. This means that an antioxidant is any substance that is able to neutralize free radicals. That's lucky for us, because it means that lots of substances, and especially many nutrients found in food, can act as antioxidants. This is a partial list.

Enzymes found in the body
- Superoxide dismutase
- Glutathione peroxidase

Vitamins
- Vitamin A
- Vitamin E
- Vitamin C

Minerals
- Selenium
- Zinc
- Copper

Phytonutrients:
- Many different types including carotenoids, phenolic compounds, and organosulfur compounds.

Proteins
- Glutathione
- Alpha-lipoic acid

Co-enzymes
- CoQ10

Foods Rich In Antioxidants

While it seems like acai berries are getting all the press, you don't need exotic or new "superfoods" to find great sources of antioxidants. From strawberries to pinto beans to cinnamon, there are plenty of great options that you've probably been eating all along.

Top Food Sources Of Antioxidants In The American Diet*

SPICES (per 100 grams)	◆ Cloves, ground ◆ Oregano leaf, dried ◆ Ginger, ground ◆ Cinnamon, ground ◆ Turmeric powder ◆ Basil leaf, dried ◆ Curry powder ◆ Paprika ◆ Chili powder ◆ Parsley, dried

VEGETABLES (per standard serving size)	◆ Artichokes, prepared ◆ Cabbage, red cooked ◆ Spinach, frozen ◆ Potatoes, red, cooked ◆ Potatoes, white, cooked ◆ Sweet potatoes, baked ◆ Broccoli rabe, cooked ◆ Peppers, red, cooked ◆ Broccoli, cooked ◆ Pinto beans

*Excludes juices or processed foods containing added antioxidants

Top Food Sources Of Antioxidants In The American Diet*

FRUITS (per standard serving size)	• Blackberries • Strawberries • Cranberries • Raspberries • Blueberries • Sour cherries • Prunes • Pineapple • Oranges • Black plums

OTHER: NUTS, SEEDS, AND BEVERAGES (per standard serving size)	• Walnuts • Coffee • Pecans • Chocolate, baking, unsweetened • Wine, red • Chocolates, dark • Molasses, dark • Iced tea, brewed, unsweetened

*Excludes juices or processed foods containing added antioxidants

*Adapted from data in/ reprinted with permission:
Halvorsen BL, Carlsen MH, Phillips KM, Bøhn SK, Holte K, Jacobs DR, Blomhoff R. Content of redox-active compounds (ie, antioxidants) in foods consumed in the United States. The American journal of clinical nutrition. 2006 Jul 1;84(1):95-135, by permission of Oxford University Press.

Quercetin, Ellagic Acid, Resveratrol, And Others: Powerful Phytonutrients

While you hear a lot about vitamins and minerals such as vitamin C, beta-carotene, and selenium, there are other compounds that also function as powerful antioxidants. Compounds that have been isolated from foods, tested in the lab, and found to have powerful disease-fighting abilities. Compounds with names such as polyphenols, glucosinolates, flavonoids, and others.

These are all phytonutrients, and they pack an impressive punch, with antioxidant, anti-inflammatory, and other benefits.

Phytonutrients Protect Plants, And They Protect You

Phytonutrients are compounds that are naturally found in plants. They're not essential (in the way that vitamins are), but the more we learn about their properties, the more important they seem to be in maintaining health and fighting disease. These compounds protect plants from the sun, heat, insects, and other threats. They also act to protect the plants from the oxidative stress that results from photosynthesis. That's why these compounds function as great antioxidants.

The more we study these compounds, the more we find that they have other powers also: fighting inflammation, promoting detoxification enzymes, and others. And when you eat these plants, you're eating the same protective chemicals.

Three major categories of phytonutrients are carotenoids, polyphenols, and organosulfur compounds. (There are more categories.)

These include a wide variety of different chemical compounds. There are thousands of polyphenolic compounds alone.

While you may hear about certain foods as great sources of certain phytonutrients, it's important to remember that one plant, literally, may contain hundreds of different compounds, including compounds from different classes.

Research has shown that synergy comes into play also, with different compounds acting together to produce stronger benefits. This provides yet another reason to focus on the benefits of foods as opposed to just single nutrients.

PHYTONUTRIENTS

Category	Specific Type	Found In
Organosulfur compounds	• Glucosinolates (Indoles, Isothiocyanates)	• Broccoli, Brussels sprouts, cauliflower, cabbage
	• Allylic sulfur compounds	• Garlic, onions
Carotenoids	• Beta-carotene	• Carrots, sweet potatoes, spinach
	• Lycopene	• Tomatoes, watermelon
	• Lutein and zeaxanthin	• Spinach, kale, summer/winter squash
Polyphenols	• Flavonoids (Flavonols, Flavones, Flavanols, Flavanones, Anthocyanidins, Isoflavonoids)	• Onions, apples, celery, thyme, basil, tea, oranges, lemons, cherries, grapes, soybeans
	• Stilbenes (Resveratrol)	• Grapes, red wine, peanuts
	• Tannins	• Tea, coffee, red wine, grapes
	• Diferuloyl methanes	• Turmeric
	• Phenolic acids (Hydroxy-cinnamic acids, Hydroxy-benzoic acids)	• Blueberries, cherries, coffee, wheat, pomegranate
	• Lignans	• Flaxseeds, sesame seeds
Other	• Chlorophylls • Enzymes • Other	• Spinach, parsley, arugula

CHAPTER 13
ANTI-INFLAMMATORY FOODS

The foods that are naturally rich in antioxidants are the same foods that form the basis for an anti-inflammatory diet. That's important for your skin, and it's important for your health.

Inflammation is the body's defense and repair process. You need the system to work quickly and effectively, and then you need the system to stand down once the threat is over.

The system, unfortunately, doesn't always work the way that it should. In some cases the entire system stays on high alert, even once the threat is removed. We call that chronic inflammation, and it's known to be harmful to many different organ systems.

There are a number of ways that you can fight chronic inflammation. One of the major ways is by eating the right foods.

Acute Inflammation:
Your Body's Defense and Repair System

When you cut your skin, your body's immune system springs into action. One of the key players in your immune system are your white blood cells, and when these are activated, they start to produce different chemicals that act as messengers. These messengers include substances known as cytokines, prostaglandins, leukotrienes, and others, and they help coordinate the body's repair process and activate the other key players in your immune system.

This repair process is what we call acute inflammation.

Think of a cut, and think of how it heals. The redness, swelling, and pain that you experience are all signs of this repair process. Once the wound is healed, the process of inflammation subsides, and your skin returns to normal.

That's acute inflammation, and it's a necessary and normal process.

Inflammation Out of Control

In some cases, though, the process of inflammation just doesn't turn off. The immune cells keep working, and the chemical messengers keep circulating in our body's tissues and in our bloodstream.

This is known as chronic inflammation, and it's a problem.

Chronic inflammation is essentially your body's defense and repair system out of control. It may start with one small trigger (an injury, an infection, an unknown trigger), but by the time your out-of-control force has done its damage, you're left with a much bigger problem. In fact, chronic inflammation is a major factor in the development of heart disease, some types of cancer, and some types of dementia. Chronic inflammation can lead to damage and breakdown of the body's tissues, which can accelerate aging. Some experts call this "inflammaging."

Which brings up an important question. Why would the body's normal repair process (acute inflammation) start to rage out of control (chronic inflammation)? Research has found that certain factors can act as a trigger for chronic inflammation. For example, cigarette smoke can cause chronic inflammation of the bronchial passages, while infection with the human papilloma virus can cause chronic inflammation of the cervical tissues.

The Way You Live Your Life Can Either Fight Inflammation Or Trigger Inflammation

Certain lifestyle factors can also trigger chronic inflammation. Luckily, those same lifestyle factors can be turned around to fight off chronic inflammation.

Fight inflammation	Worsen inflammation
• Regular exercise • Strong social ties • Strong coping strategies • The right foods	• A sedentary lifestyle • Social isolation • Chronic stress • The wrong foods

The right foods can fight chronic inflammation.

Scientists have done extensive research on foods and their effects on chronic inflammation. What they've discovered is that diet plays a central role in regulating chronic inflammation.

Scientific Research

One of the ways to measure chronic inflammation is to measure the levels of certain compounds in the bloodstream. We call these inflammatory biomarkers, and they tell us about levels of inflammation in the body. One of these markers is called C-reactive protein (CRP). Studies have found that when CRP levels are elevated, your risk of serious medical events, such as stroke or heart attack, can go up by as much as 400%.

How can you bring down levels of CRP? A major way is with the right foods.

What Are The Foods That Fight Off Inflammation?

We actually have a lot of data to answer this question. Laboratory, animal, and human studies have looked at the effects of different foods and nutrients on inflammatory biomarkers (substances in your bloodstream that indicate the level of inflammation in your body).

- Researchers looked at over 1900 of these studies.
- They looked at the effects of many different foods and nutrients on 6 major biomarkers of inflammation.
- If a food or nutrient increased levels of IL-1B, IL-6, TNF-alpha, or CRP, or decreased levels of IL-4 or IL-10, then it was acting to worsen inflammation. If it did the opposite, it was fighting inflammation.
- The researchers combined the results of the different research studies. They then created a score called the dietary inflammatory index (DII).
- The DII tells us whether a food is anti-inflammatory (fights inflammation) or pro-inflammatory (worsens inflammation).

* Shivappa N, Steck SE, Hurley TG, Hussey JR, Hébert JR. Designing and developing a literature-derived, population-based dietary inflammatory index. Public Health Nutrition. 2014 Aug;17:1689-96.

Summary of Foods That Fight Inflammation

Categories	Examples
Plant foods rich in nutrients and fiber	• Vegetables • Legumes
Carbohydrates rich in nutrients and fiber	• Whole grains
Herbs & Spices	• Turmeric, black pepper, oregano, rosemary
Healthy Fats	• Omega-3 fats

Summary of Foods That Worsen Inflammation

Categories	Examples
Processed foods and beverages high in calories but low in nutrients	• Sugar sweetened drinks • Sugar sweetened foods
Carbohydrates high in calories but low in nutrients	• White flour • White rice
Processed meats	• Hotdogs
Unhealthy fats	• Fatty red meats

Are these foods helpful purely because they're anti-inflammatory? We don't know, because these foods have other benefits, such as high levels of antioxidants.

(Emphasizing again the point that a single food can have lots of different beneficial effects on the body.) What we do know is that people who eat a diet based on anti-inflammatory foods have a lower risk for a number of chronic diseases.

From turmeric to anthocyanidins to selenium, the research on anti-inflammatory foods has been very wide-ranging. That's very helpful, because it provides us with more data points. The table below provides an estimate of anti-inflammatory power, starting with some of the strongest foods and nutrients.

ANTI-INFLAMMATORY FOODS AND NUTRIENTS

ANTI-INFLAMMATORY FOODS	Turmeric, green/black tea, ginger, garlic, onion, alcohol (moderate portion), saffron, pepper, thyme/oregano
ANTI-INFLAMMATORY MACRO AND MICRONUTRIENTS	Fiber, magnesium, vitamin D, omega 3 fatty acids, vitamin C, vitamin E, vitamin A, vitamin B6, zinc, niacin, selenium, folic acid
ANTI-INFLAMMATORY PHYTONUTRIENTS	Flavones, isoflavones, beta carotene, flavonols, flavan-3-ol, flavonones, anthocyanidins

Skin Saving Foods Often Have Many Superpowers

The foods that are naturally rich in antioxidants are the same foods that have powerful anti-inflammatory benefits. But their benefits don't stop there: the foods in these two chapters, and in the chapters that follow, have multiple superpowers.

Broccoli, for example, is a great source of the antioxidant vitamin C. It's also a detox food: it's a great source of phytonutrients called glycosinolates that provide powerful detoxification abilities. It's also a great source of fiber.

Here's a small sampling of some of the other skin saving nutrients and anti-aging properties that these foods provide:

•**Beta-carotene and Vitamin A/ Cell Renewal**: Beta-carotene is a strong antioxidant, but it's also what we call a provitamin: the body is able to convert it to another form. Beta-carotene is converted to vitamin A, an important skin nutrient that ensures cell turnover and skin renewal. (The anti-aging prescription cream tretinoin is a form of topical vitamin A.) Strong sources include many red/orange fruits and vegetables, along with green leafy vegetables.

•**Iron/Necessary for Hair Growth:** Hair follicle cells are some of the most rapidly dividing cells in the body, and one of the important enzymes in this process requires iron. For patients with unexplained hair loss, dermatologists recommend blood tests to check levels of iron stored in the body. Food sources include plant-based sources, especially beans, lentils, and spinach, as well as meat sources, such as sardines, salmon, and chicken.

•**Niacin/Energy for DNA Repair:** The body uses niacin (vitamin B3) to produce nicotinamide, which has been shown to enhance DNA repair. In an experimental trial, volunteers given nicotinamide for 1 year developed fewer skin cancers. Strong sources include peanuts, sunflower seeds, and tuna.

•Polyphenols/ Collagen Protection: Polyphenols are one of the major classes of phytonutrients, and there are thousands of them. They're divided into different categories based on their chemical structure, and as more research has been done, some have shown remarkable collagen-protecting abilities. Flavonoids are one category of polyphenols, and are mainly found in fruits, vegetables, and tea. Some of these flavonoid compounds, including luteolin, quercetin, and rutin, have shown the ability in laboratory studies to protect collagen from the damaging effects of sugar. They've done this by inhibiting the production of AGEs (advanced glycation end products), the sugar-protein compounds that act to weaken collagen. Strong sources include fruits and vegetables such as onions, cauliflower, apples, celery, figs, and asparagus.

CHAPTER 14
HERBS AND SPICES

♦ Why are herbs and spices so important for healthy skin?

♦ How can I consume more?

Top Antioxidant-Rich Spices and Herbs

♦ CLOVES	♦ OREGANO	♦ NUTMEG
♦ MINT	♦ THYME	♦ GINGER
♦ ALLSPICE	♦ ROSEMARY	♦ DILL
♦ CINNAMON	♦ SAFFRON	♦ BASIL
	♦ SAGE	

You <u>could</u> keep eating your regular brown rice bowl. The one with brown rice, beans, and vegetables. It's packed full of healthy goodness. But you could also choose to power it up even more. You would start by sautéeing the vegetables with garlic, ginger, and onions. You would ramp up the flavor with ground cinnamon, cloves, and cumin seeds. You would add in plenty of chopped cilantro for more flavor, texture, color, and phytonutrient punch.

Now you've got a rice bowl that's more interesting and more flavorful. And one that packs in way more power. (The recipe for this power bowl is found in Chapter 30: Skin Saving Salads.)

While vegetables get all the glory, spices and herbs are also very valuable sources of phytonutrients. I think of them as "triple threats".

That's because spices and herbs combat the three major forces that challenge your skin:

- They're a great source of antioxidants.
- They act as anti-inflammatory agents.
- Some combat the process of glycation and collagen cross-linking. Some may even act to lower   blood sugar levels.

Spices and herbs have other benefits as well. They exhibit antimicrobial effects, and their rich supply of phytonutrients means that they provide benefits for other organ systems as well.

SPICES

Spices can be obtained from a number of different plants (either woody or non-woody plants). When you think of spices, think "seed to bark".

- **Root-like stems**: Turmeric, ginger
- **Seeds**: Cumin, cardamom
- **Bark**: Cinnamon
- **Berries**: Allspice, peppercorns
- **Flowers**: Saffron (stigma), cloves (buds)

Spices are dried, and you can purchase them either whole (such as whole cloves or cumin seeds) or ground (such as ground cumin).

HERBS

Herbs are the leafy parts of plants with non-woody stems. Basil and mint are some of the classic examples. Other common (and powerful) herbs are cilantro, rosemary, oregano, dill, thyme, and parsley.

You can purchase herbs either fresh or dried, and both types have notable health benefits.

THE POWER OF SPICE

As a group, herbs and spices contain thousands of phytochemicals. They're especially known for their high concentrations of polyphenols, a group of phytonutrients known for their antioxidant powers. As a bonus, drying an herb or spice helps to concentrate those polyphenols. This means that your spice rack can add an impressive nutritional punch to your meal.

The nice thing about herbs and spices is that you can use a variety throughout the day, added to just about every snack and meal. That ensures a variety of phytonutrients, provided via small, regular doses.

Cinnamon is one example of an easy-to-use spice with impressive powers. Cinnamon pairs well with both sweet and savory dishes. It's easy to add to pancake batter, AND it's frequently used in Indian cuisine (it's one of the main ingredients in some garam masala/Indian spice mix recipes). Cinnamon is high in antioxidants, it has anti-inflammatory properties, and it's been shown to reduce the production of collagen-damaging AGEs. In some people, it may even reduce blood sugar levels, in doses as low as ¼ to ½ teaspoon daily. Laboratory and animal studies suggest that it may do this by increasing the sensitivity of our insulin receptors.

The table at the start of this chapter is just a sample of the many herbs and spices that provide important health benefits. As more are researched, we're likely to uncover many more. Although I've listed some of the top examples below, it's difficult to actually rank the most powerful ones. (This is due to differences in species, parts of the plants studied, time of harvest, and research methods used.) This is just a sample; there are many, many more with the same benefits.

The Power of Spice: Research Studies

- **Anti-inflammatory Powers:** Turmeric, ginger, garlic, saffron, pepper, thyme, oregano, rosemary, parsley

- **Rich Source of Antioxidants:** In a USDA study of the top 50 antioxidant-rich foods (per 100 gm weight), the top 5 five were dried spices: clove, oregano, ginger, cinnamon, turmeric

- **Antioxidant Powers:** In another study, cloves, cinnamon, and oregano scored highest, with sage, thyme, rosemary, bay, and mint also with high levels

Spices and Glycation

- Multiple herbs and spices act to limit glycation, as well as the damage from glycation.
- Some have been shown to help reduce the production of AGEs, including cinnamon, cloves, oregano, and allspice.
- Other foods that reduce AGE formation include ginger, garlic, and green tea.
- Some herbs and spices have also been shown to act after AGEs have formed, by reducing the damage they cause.
- Some spices may even help reduce blood sugar in the first place, including cinnamon, ginger, turmeric, fenugreek, cumin seeds, mustard seeds, coriander seeds, and cloves.

CHAPTER 15
POWER CARBS

♦ What are power carbs?
♦ Why are they important for healthy skin?
♦ How can I consume more?

SOME TOP SOURCES OF POWER CARBS

INTACT WHOLE GRAINS	Whole oats, brown rice, quinoa, millet, buckwheat, wild rice, farro, bulgur, wheatberries
FOODS MADE WITH WHOLE GRAINS	Whole wheat bread, whole wheat tortillas, rye bread
LEGUMES	Lentils (red, green, brown, other), beans (black, kidney, pinto, garbanzo, edamame, cannellini, other), peas
VEGETABLES	Sweet potatoes, spaghetti squash, butternut squash

Carbohydrates are a major macronutrient, and they're critical to your health. But for years now, there's been a raging debate in certain circles. "Are carbs good or bad for you?"

Are Carbs Good Or Bad For You?
(What do you mean by carbs? And who are you?)

What do you mean by carbs? Carbohydrates, affectionately referred to as carbs, can be tricky. The wrong kind, and too much, and you have major health problems. On the other hand, you need carbs in your diet. You need the right kind, and the right amount, in order to fuel your brain and your body.

Carbohydrates provide energy for your body and brain. The fiber in some carbs also promotes a healthy gut.

Carbohydrates include sugars, starch, and fiber. Your body needs sugars and starches because they're a great source of energy: when you digest them, they break down into glucose and enter the bloodstream to provide quick energy.

The fiber in many carbohydrate-containing foods is also very important. Fiber doesn't have any calories because you don't digest it, but fiber maintains a healthy gut and it supports the growth of good gut microbes. Those microbes impact your gut health, your immune system, and your metabolism.

There's a whole lot of different carbs that you could be eating. (And that you need to be eating, because carbs are a basic macronutrient.) But there's a big difference in the carbs that are out there, and there's a big difference in the way that they affect your body.

Not all carbs are created equal: when judging a carb, think about quality, quantity, and the company that it keeps.

When you look at a food that's sitting on your plate, you need to know a few things before you eat it. You should judge a carb by three things:

- Quality: Power carbs provide more nutrients
- Quantity: Portion sizes are critical
- The company that it keeps: Eating carbs in the company of fiber, protein, and fat helps limit sugar spikes

Quality: Power carbs are naturally rich in fiber, vitamins, minerals, and phytonutrients. Some even contain protein and fat.

When you're choosing your carbs, think power. Power carbs are sources of carbohydrates that are naturally rich in a whole host of powerful nutrients. These foods are naturally rich in fiber, vitamins, minerals, phytonutrients, and sometimes protein and fat. I'm including that term "naturally rich" because fortified processed foods (such as processed cereals with 10 added vitamins and minerals) just aren't able to provide all of the powerful nutrients that the original foods would.

These nutrients provide power: many have antioxidant and anti-inflammatory properties, while fiber slows down digestion, stabilizes blood sugar levels, and promotes a healthy gut.

One experiment found calorie-burning benefits with a diet rich in whole grains.

Two groups of volunteers ate similar diets for 6 weeks, with one big difference: one group ate mainly whole grains, while the other group ate mainly refined grains. This one change resulted in an estimated higher calorie burn of 92 calories/day in the whole grain group.

Quantity: Watch Out For Serving Sizes

You need enough carbs to provide energy (because they're a preferred fuel source for the body), but not so much that you're flooding your bloodstream and liver with excess glucose. This is true for all types of carbs. If you eat too much brown rice, you can still send your blood sugar soaring. And for many carbs, it's really easy to consume 2 or 3 (or even more) serving sizes without even realizing it. (Try it: measure out a ½ cup serving of pasta and compare that to what you might normally put on your plate.)

This brings up another important point: some people can handle larger quantities of carbs than others. There's more on the research behind carb sensitivity in Chapter 18: Stop Sugar Spikes.

Balanced Meals: Eat Your Carbs Alongside Fiber, Protein, And Fat

While the ideal carbs contain fiber (and sometimes protein), it's also important to eat these carbs in the right company.

A healthy plate emphasizes balance. Half the plate should be covered in produce (lots of vegetables), while the other half is split between healthy sources of carbs and protein.

That protein balances out the carbs and slows down the release of glucose into the bloodstream. A little bit of fat with your meal does the same. Measurements of blood sugar levels confirm the benefits of balanced meals: adding fiber-rich foods (such as black beans and chickpeas) or healthy protein sources to carb-heavy meals improves the blood sugar response.

Power Carbs Help Maintain Youthful Skin

- They promote slow steady levels of blood glucose, as opposed to skin-aging sugar spikes.
- They're a great source of prebiotic fiber, which supports the growth of skin-protective good gut microbes.
- They're a great source of vitamins and minerals, such as the antioxidant vitamin E (found in whole wheat) and the anti-inflammatory mineral zinc (found in red kidney beans).
- They're also a great source of a huge variety of phytonutrients, such as the carotenoids in sweet potatoes and the anthocyanidins in black beans.

Sources of Carbohydrates

When you think of carbs, you may picture bread and pasta. There are plenty of other sources, though. These include power carbs (intact grains, whole grain foods, vegetables, lentils, beans, fruits) and other foods (such as milk). Other sources include empty carbs, so named because they're lacking in nutrients. This group includes refined carbohydrates, such as white bread and white pasta, and processed foods with added sugars.

Why Whole Foods Are Better Than Refined Foods

You're at your favorite Chinese restaurant. As the waiter asks you what type of rice you want, you start to wonder: is brown rice really that much better for you than white rice?

Simply put, yes. Whole grains pack in way more power.

Think about wheat. A wheat plant is a tall grass, and the seed of that grass is called a wheat kernel. That kernel is made up of 3 main parts.

Wheat Bran: The bran is the outer layer, and it's high in fiber. (That's the bran in bran cereal.) Wheat bran is high in fiber, and it's also high in nutrients, especially minerals and B vitamins. In fact, the bran provides most of the B vitamins that are found in wheat.

Wheat Germ: Wheat germ is found at the center. (That's the wheat germ that you sprinkle on your cereal.) This is the part of the seed that can grow into a new plant, and it's high in vitamins, minerals, and fatty acids. These are powerful nutrients. Vitamin E, for example, is a powerful antioxidant, while the minerals magnesium, zinc, copper, and selenium have antioxidant, anti-inflammatory, and other properties.

The Carb-Heavy Endosperm: The largest part of the seed is called the endosperm, and it provides energy for growing plants. That means that it's mainly carbohydrates, with a much smaller amount of vitamins and minerals.

When you eat intact wheat kernels, you're consuming all of this nutritional power.

When you grind down wheat kernels, you end up with snow white flour, but you lose the bran and the germ.

As you start grinding down those wheat kernels, you lose the bran and germ. By the time you're done, you're left with snow white flour, which keeps well on a shelf. But isn't so great for your health.

This refining process is why, when you eat a slice of white bread, you're mainly just eating carbs. You've refined away most of the nutrients and the fiber.

Are whole grains really that much better than refined grains?

Absolutely. If you look at processed, unenriched white bread, it only contains 2% of the niacin levels found in whole grain bread.

Although you can add back in some nutrients, you can't add back in ALL of the vitamins, minerals and phytonutrients that you lose during the refining process.

Although manufacturers advertise "10 added vitamins and minerals", it's important to note that enriched white flour can never add in the same number of nutrients that are found in whole wheat. While enriched white flour does add back in B vitamins and iron, it doesn't add back in vitamin E, magnesium, manganese, selenium, and zinc (and that's just for starters).

CHAPTER 16
POWER FATS

- ♦ What are power fats?
- ♦ Why are they so important for healthy skin?
- ♦ How can I consume more?

SOME TOP SOURCES OF POWER FATS

MONOUNSATURATED FATTY ACIDS (MUFAS)	Avocados, cashews, almonds, hazelnuts, peanut butter, pumpkin seeds, olive oil, canola oil
OMEGA-3 FATTY ACIDS (OMEGA-3 PUFAS)	Walnuts, flaxseeds, flaxseed oil Fatty fish, including herring, mackerel, salmon, sardines, trout, tuna

Avocado toast. Roasted salmon. Apple slices with creamy almond butter. These foods are enjoying a wave of popularity, even though a few years ago their fat content would have been a concern. No longer. It's now known that the right types of fats, in the right amounts, can promote overall health. These fats can also help maintain youthful skin. That's because research has found that certain fats can protect against the 3 major forces that damage your skin: oxidation, inflammation, and glycation.

Certain Fats Provide Skin-Saving Nutrients

The right fats can protect against free radical damage (combat oxidative stress). The right fats can also calm down inflammation (combat inflammation). In the right amounts, some fats can also help stabilize blood sugar levels (combat glycation). This means that the right fats, in the right amounts, and in the right balance, can be important skin saving nutrients.

When Choosing Fats, Think Quality, Quantity, And Balance

Fat is a major macronutrient, and it's essential for our health. Our bodies need us to eat fat, because those fatty acids are needed for normal growth and development. They also help maintain the flexibility and function of our cell membranes, and they serve as building materials for the lipids that act to reinforce our skin barrier. Fat is also necessary to absorb the fat-soluble vitamins A, D, E, and K.

You need to eat fat for another reason as well: it helps you feel full. It also helps to slow down the digestion of carbohydrates, which means it helps stabilize blood sugar levels.

But as most of us have heard, there are healthy fats and unhealthy fats. Eat the wrong type, or too much of any type, and you increase your risk of obesity, heart disease, and other medical conditions.

In terms of food sources of fats, it's important to remember that most foods contain a combination of different fats. Canola oil, for example, contains mostly monounsaturated fat, although it also contains a sizeable proportion of polyunsaturated fat. When experts talk about food sources of fat, they tend to just refer to the most common type of fat found in that food.

Monounsaturated Fats (MUFAs) May Increase Skin Elasticity And Protect Against Signs Of Photoaging

Great sources of MUFAs include avocados, peanut butter, olives, and olive oil. Research indicates that they may raise levels of HDL, the "good" cholesterol.

MUFAs also have demonstrated skin benefits.

In one study, participants who reported a higher intake of MUFAs from olive oil were graded by trained observers as having fewer wrinkles and dark spots.

In another study, individuals reporting higher intakes of MUFAs displayed more elasticity in their skin.

Omega-3 Polyunsaturated Fats (PUFAs) Have Powerful Anti-Inflammatory Effects

ESSENTIAL FATTY ACIDS PUFAs are essential fatty acids. These can't be synthesized by the body, so we need to consume them via foods. The two families of PUFAs are omega-3 fatty acids and omega-6 fatty acids. You need both types in your diet, but the balance between the two is very important.

OMEGA-3 FATTY ACIDS Omega-3s in particular are well-known for their ability to help fight inflammation. They also help support the immune system and maintain a healthy skin barrier.

There are 3 main types of omega-3s. Alpha-linolenic acid is found in plant foods such as flaxseeds and walnuts. Your body converts ALA to the two other types of omega-3s: EHA (eicosapentaenoic acid) and DHA (docosahexaenoic acid), although this process in our body isn't very efficient. Fatty fish, on the other hand, contain EHA and DHA already pre-formed (fish make these from the algae in their diet). This means that fatty fish such as salmon and sardines are great sources of these powerful omega-3s.

ANTIOXIDANT AND ANTI-INFLAMMATORY PROPERTIES In dermatology, omega-3 fatty acids have been shown to protect against oxidation and calm down inflammation.

> Volunteers consumed EHA (an omega-3 fatty acid) every day for 3 months.
>
> At the end of that time, their skin showed less of a sunburn response to UV radiation. Their skin and immune cells even showed less DNA damage.

Omega-3s have been studied in the treatment of multiple inflammatory skin diseases, with promising preliminary research in acne, eczema, psoriasis, and other skin conditions. Because of these promising initial results, more research has been called for.

Quantity: No Trans Fats, Careful with Saturated Fats, and Unsaturated Fats in Moderation

The general rules for fats are these: No trans fats at all, since they're so harmful. Be careful with saturated fats, especially while research is sorting out how much and what type (plant vs animal sources) can be incorporated into a healthy diet.

Which brings us to the power fats. Since nuts are so good for you, is it OK to just snack on some roasted walnuts every time you walk by the bowl on your desk? (You can probably guess the answer.)

The answer is (you guessed it) moderation. Yes, nuts are good for you, but too much and you'll have problems.

Of the three macronutrients (protein, carbohydrates, and fats), fat is the most calorically dense. That means it's really easy to overdo it.

The guiding principles when it comes to consuming power fats are these:

- Focus on fats in the form of whole foods
- That means foods such as nuts, seeds, olives, avocados, and fatty fish
- But even with whole food fats, you need to watch out for serving sizes. And as with carbs, some people may need to be more cautious with their fat intake
- It's very easy to overdo it, especially with nuts and seeds. A serving size of almonds, for example, is one ounce, which translates to about 23 almonds
- Vegetable oils (even extra virgin olive oil) are processed and very calorie dense. Depending on your calorie needs, you should generally limit your intake to 1-2 tablespoons of oil a day.
- That oil should be INSTEAD of other fat sources

- 1 tablespoon of olive oil contains about 120 calories and 14 grams of fat. That's why, when you're cooking, don't glug your olive oil: instead, measure it by the teaspoon/tablespoon
- The same goes for almond butter: creamy and tasty, but very calorie dense, so pull out the tablespoon

The Right Balance Between Omega-3s and Omega-6s is Important

Why is salmon so popular while corn oil is falling out of favor? It's because of the balance between omega-3s and omega-6s in the American diet.

PUFAs are considered power fats, but with this type of fat you have to consider more than just the quality and quantity of the fat. You also have to think about whether your PUFA food sources are in the right balance. That means that you need to eat the right balance of omega-3 fatty acids to omega-6 fatty acids.

While omega-3s get all the press because of their potent anti-inflammatory properties, omega-6 fatty acids are also important to include in your diet. However, you usually don't need to make much of an effort in the United States to include them, because they're already so prevalent in the American food supply. They're found in commonly used vegetable oils such as corn and soybean oil. They're also commonly found in American meat, eggs, and dairy, including our milk and butter. That's because American cows and chickens are commonly fed with seeds (high in omega-6 FAs) as opposed to the grass (high in omega-3 FAs) that these animals would eat in nature.

In fact, this change in the American food supply has been suggested by some experts as a major cause of our increasing levels of inflammatory disease. In the last decades, our dietary intake of omega-3s has gone down, while our intake of omega-6s has gone up.

Traditionally, people would consume about equal amounts of omega-3s and omega6s. Now it's estimated that omega-6s are consumed in vastly higher amounts than omega-3s, with an estimated ratio of over 20:1.

Why is that believed to be a problem? Omega-3s compete with omega-6s during certain steps of the inflammation process. When there's the right balance (with enough omega-3s) the inflammatory system produces chemicals that aren't as inflammatory or that are even anti-inflammatory.

The importance of consuming the right balance of fats may even impact skin cancer.

In one study, mice were exposed to a hefty dose of UV radiation, and all developed skin cancers. Researchers wanted to see if a change in their diets would be enough to change this.

They fed one group of mice a diet high in omega-3s, and the other group a diet high in omega-6s.

This one change had a big impact: the omega-3 group developed fewer skin cancers, while the omega-6 group actually developed more.

In practice, this means that you may need to make an active effort to consume more omega-3s in your diet—especially since the American food supply isn't geared around them. Whether that's seeking out plant-based sources (ground flaxseeds, walnuts) or fish-based sources (salmon, albacore tuna, sardines), finding a few extra recipes that incorporate these foods will pay off in a powerful nutrient boost.

CHAPTER 17
PREBIOTICS AND PROBIOTICS

♦ What are prebiotics?
♦ Why are they so important for healthy skin?
♦ How can I consume more?

PREBIOTIC FOODS

VEGETABLES	Artichokes, asparagus, leafy greens, onions, jicama, soybeans, legumes
FRUITS	Bananas, berries
GRAINS	Whole wheat, oats, barley
NUTS AND SEEDS	Almonds, walnuts, flaxseeds
OTHER	Garlic

Prebiotic foods and probiotic foods help maintain a healthy gut, and research has shown that this helps maintain healthy skin. It's especially important to ensure that your gut contains "good" microbes. The major way to do that is by eating the right foods.

- For healthy skin, you need a healthy gut.
- A healthy gut contains plenty of "good" microbes. Our gut actually contains trillions of microbes. In a healthy gut, the good guys ("good microbes") far outnumber the bad guys ("harmful germs" or pathogens).
- These good microbes work hard to keep us healthy. They also produce substances that help fight inflammation.
- To help these good microbes flourish in our gut, we have to feed them the right kinds of foods. Foods that encourage the growth of good microbes are called prebiotics.
- Prebiotic foods include foods that are naturally rich in plant fibers, especially fruits, vegetables, and whole grains. Other phytonutrients found in fruits and vegetables (such as polyphenols), and even certain fats, can help promote the growth of good microbes.
- You can also consume good bacteria and other microbes, In the form of probiotic foods or supplements. (Although it's very important to keep feeding them prebiotics.)

Good Bacteria And Bad Bacteria: Why Some Germs Are Our Friends And Protectors

Your body is covered in germs. Don't be alarmed: that's normal. In fact, it's a good thing.

Your skin, mouth, nose, and other body parts are covered in germs. But the part of your body that contains the most germs is actually inside of you: your gut (in medical terms, the gastrointestinal tract).

These germs, known as microbes, have important roles to play in keeping us healthy.

There are actually trillions of microbes on (and inside) your body. These microbes include bacteria, viruses, and other groups.

- This entire community of microbes is known as the microbiota.
- These microbes and the genes (genetic material) that they contain are called the microbiome.

You may have heard of the microbiome in medical news, because research has now found a strong link between a healthy gut and our overall health. To start with, the gut is actually considered an important part of the immune system. In one study, certain strains of gut microbes regulated the expression of genes that impacted the immune system.

That's important, because if your immune system hasn't been trained properly, it starts to overreact to everything--foods, pollen, and sometimes even the cells of our own body. People with an over-reacting immune system may develop allergies and sometimes even autoimmune diseases.

It's not just allergic diseases, either. Studies have linked the gut microbiome to obesity, depression, and other chronic illnesses.

Research has found that your gut health impacts your skin health. A healthy gut microbiome helps to maintain skin hydration, counter skin inflammation, and fight off the damaging effects of free radicals.

How Good Gut Microbes Help Us: Teachers, Policemen, And Factory Workers

In a healthy gut, there may be some pathogens (harmful bacteria), but they're far outnumbered by the good guys: the good microbes. What do these "good gut microbes" do?

> Your gut microbes act as teachers, as policemen, and as factory workers. They've been shown to help train our immune system, fight off the harmful germs that sometimes find their way into our digestive system, and even actively help to break down and digest our food.

In fact, we need these helpful microbes to digest many of our foods. The human body alone doesn't produce all of the enzymes needed to digest all types of foods. Different microbes contain different enzymes. These enzymes are critical in the digestion of certain foods, such as fiber-rich vegetables. They help break down these fibers and extract the nutrients. They help in another way also: they take that fiber and use it to produce helpful substances.

When Your Microbes Are Well Fed, They Really Try To Help You

When you feed your microbes fiber, they start digesting and fermenting that fiber. In the process, they produce some very helpful substances. These substances are called short chain fatty acids. There are different ones, including acetate, butyrate, and propionate. Research has found that these short chain fatty acids (SCFAs) help us in a number of ways. SCFAs help fight inflammation. They also help protect the lining of our gut, which may help protect us from allergies and infections.

Good Microbes Are Picky Eaters, But They Love Fiber: Why A Diet Rich In Fruits, Vegetables, And Whole Grains Is So Good For Your Gut

When it comes to your health, it's always important to evaluate the research and then think about the actions that you can take. In this case, knowing that these good microbes are so important for our health, how can we make sure that they grow and flourish in our gut?

One major way is by feeding them the right kinds of foods.

Research has shown that all of us have very distinct communities of microbes living on and inside of us. In other words, your germs are different than my germs.

Studies have shown that this is due to many different factors. Genetics plays a role, as does your age and other medical conditions. The medications you take play a role as well. For example, we know that while taking broad-spectrum antibiotics (such as that Z-Pak for your sinus infection) can eradicate harmful, infection-causing bacteria, they can also kill off some of the good microbes.

But genetics, age, and medical conditions aren't the only factors. A major factor is your diet.

Less Processed Foods And More Whole Foods: Why It's So Important

One of the most important ways that you can influence the health of your gut is through your diet.

Your microbes eat what you eat. And they can be a picky lot. A diet high in added sugar and refined carbohydrates can cause some of your good microbes to die off. A diet rich in whole foods, on the other hand, helps them flourish.

Let's start with the research. The foods that you eat are so important to the composition of your gut microbiome that you can see changes after just one day. In one study, researchers found that switching from a fiber-rich, plant-based diet to a more Westernized diet, high in sugar and high in fat, led to changes in the gut microbes after just ONE day.

The changes go the other way, too. Researchers have found that if you start to eat more fiber, your gut starts to contain more of the good microbes.

Good microbes love to eat fiber. And they're really good at it too. You actually need the help of these microbes to digest certain types of fiber. Without these microbes living in our gut, we just can't digest certain fibers. That can result in pain, along with constipation and/or diarrhea. In fact, it's believed that some cases of irritable bowel syndrome (IBS) may be due to changes in the gut resulting in a loss of the "good bacteria." An imbalance of gut microbes (loss of the good microbes with overgrowth of the "bad" ones) is known as "gut dysbiosis."

The bottom line: To help grow more of the good microbes in your gut, you have to keep feeding them fiber. And that's where prebiotics come in.

Prebiotic Foods: The Importance Of Fruits, Vegetables, And Whole Grains

To maintain a healthy gut, you need the right foods. And that means prebiotics. Prebiotics are defined as foods or substances that promote the growth of good gut microbes.

Researchers have identified lots of different foods that can be considered prebiotics. The largest category is foods that are naturally rich in plant fibers. This includes fruits, vegetables, and whole grains.

The list below is just a sampling. There are many other fruits, vegetables, and whole grains that contain prebiotic fibers. Some contain more, some contain less, but all are likely to be helpful.

- **VEGETABLES:** Artichokes, asparagus, leafy greens, onions, jicama, soybeans, legumes
- **FRUITS:** Bananas, berries
- **GRAINS:** Whole wheat, oats, barley
- **NUTS AND SEEDS:** Almonds, walnuts, flaxseeds
- **OTHER:** Garlic

> If you've been diagnosed with gut dysbiosis (or suspect it may be playing a role in your IBS), speak with your physician about how to proceed with prebiotic foods. If you don't currently have enough "good microbes", you may have difficulty digesting some of these foods, and you may need to proceed slowly.

Other Foods And Nutrients Can Help Promote The Growth Of Good Microbes

The major category of prebiotic foods are foods that are naturally rich in fiber. But research has found that other nutrients found in whole foods may also act as prebiotics. For example, many fruits and vegetables contain polyphenols. These nutrients, such as the anthocyanins that are found in red grapes and red kidney beans, are powerful antioxidants. Research has found that these polyphenols also encourage the growth of good gut microbes. Other nutrients may also act as prebiotics, such as certain fats.

Processed Foods Labeled As "High Fiber": Why Processed Fiber May Not Be The Same As The Fiber In Vegetables

You know that fiber is good for you. But that brings up an important question when you're actually in the supermarket staring at a shelf stuffed with "healthy" snack foods.

Is a "high fiber" granola bar good for you in the same way that a bowl of strawberries would be good for you?

They both contain fiber, but researchers have their suspicions about the fiber that's added to processed foods. While some granola bars may be naturally rich in fiber (due to ingredients such as lightly processed dates and nuts), other granola bars need factories to make their fiber.

Some manufacturers start with fibers, such as chicory root fiber and inulin, and then pulverize those fibers to create fiber additives. These additives are then added back to the bars.

Here's the problem: we still don't know whether our gut microbes like these processed fiber additives as much as they like the fiber found in fruits and vegetables.

Until we know for sure, I wouldn't recommend that you rely solely on "high-fiber" processed foods to feed your gut microbes. While it's possible that they may be helpful, you'll still need lots and lots of fruits, vegetables, and whole grains.

Why A Yogurt Every Day Just Isn't The Same As Eating A Wide Variety Of Prebiotic Foods:
[You Need A Variety Of Different Microbes (And Lots Of Them) For A Healthy Gut]

In a healthy gastrointestinal (GI) system, there are many, many different types of microbes. That diversity of microbes is believed to help protect against chronic conditions (I say "believed" because research is ongoing).

However, if you just eat the same few foods day after day, you're not likely to end up with a wide variety of gut microbes.

That's one of the reasons why experts always emphasize the importance of eating a wide variety of fruits, vegetables, and whole grains.

These different fruits, vegetables, and whole grains each supply a different type of plant fiber. This means that you're feeding different types of gut microbes. And that means that you're growing different gut microbes.

All of which adds up to a more diverse community of microbes residing in your gut.

The importance of gut diversity is also the reason why just eating a cup of probiotic yogurt every day just isn't enough, by itself, for a healthy gut. Many commercially available strains of yogurt contain 1 or 2, or maybe 10, different strains of bacteria. Your gut probably contains over a thousand different species of bacteria alone.

In other words, you can't just rely on a cup of probiotic yogurt every day. While that can help, it really is far more important to eat the rainbow: you need to consume a wide variety of fruits and vegetables.

Bottom Line: Foods Naturally Rich In Fiber Are Good. But How Much Fiber Are We Talking About?

The USDA recommends that women consume 25 grams of dietary fiber a day, and men 38 grams.

Between fruits, vegetables, and whole grains, you can get there. But it's not an amount that's easy to achieve if you eat the typical American diet. You may have to make a concerted effort to slowly increase your fiber intake. (In the recipe section, you'll find a number of recipes that feature foods naturally rich in fiber, such as chickpeas, bulgur, red kidney beans, black beans, and lentils.)

You also don't want to start eating that much fiber tomorrow.

If your system isn't used to that much fiber, it's important to work your way up gradually. That gives your gut microbes time to get used to digesting that much fiber. It also gives your gut microbes more time to grow and multiply in response to this great new source of their favorite food. (And if you produce a lot of gas right now when you eat beans, it's good to know that eventually your system tends to get used to the fiber in those beans.) Along with that increased fiber intake, you'll need to make sure you're drinking plenty of water.

If It's So Important That Your Gut Contain Good Microbes, Can You Eat These Good Microbes?

Yes, you can, in the form of probiotic foods and supplements consumed as part of a diet that contains plenty of prebiotics.

What Are Probiotics?

Probiotics are defined as live microorganisms (such as bacteria) which provide a health benefit when consumed in adequate amounts, such as via foods or supplements. Probiotics may benefit gut, skin, and overall health.

You may have heard probiotics referred to as "good bacteria." When you buy a carton of yogurt with "live, active cultures," you're buying probiotics.

Probiotic foods have been prized in many cultures for centuries. I met a colleague from Czechoslovakia who told me how her grandparents were adamant about eating sauerkraut every day in the winter. Friends from India tell me that when they were growing up, they were told to eat their yogurt every day because it was so good for them.

Research has now found that probiotics are indeed important for our health, and studies have started to unravel why that is.

Dermatology researchers in particular have become very interested in probiotic foods and supplements. That's because a number of clinical trials have suggested that they may help in the treatment of inflammatory skin diseases. The most evidence comes from studies of patients with atopic dermatitis (AD, also known as eczema).

Synbiotics are a combination of probiotics and prebiotics. In one summary study (combining the results of multiple trials), researchers found that synbiotics were helpful adjuncts in the treatment of AD in adults and children (over the age of 1 year), when used for at least 8 weeks, and when the probiotics combined multiple strains of bacteria.

Probiotic Foods

Probiotics may come in the form of foods or supplements. For foods, this includes a wide variety of fermented foods in which "live, active cultures" of microbes are a key component. This includes fermented dairy products (such as yogurt and kefir), fermented cabbage (such as sauerkraut and kimchi) and others (such as miso, tempeh, vinegar, other pickled vegetables, and other foods).

Probiotic Foods

BEVERAGES	Kefir (dairy), kombucha (tea), lassi (dairy)
FOODS	Fermented/ pickled vegetables, kimchi (cabbage + spices), sauerkraut (cabbage), tempeh (soy), yogurt (dairy)
FOODS/SEASONINGS	Miso (soy), vinegar (with live cultures)

Probiotic Processed Foods: More Data Needed

Are probiotic snack bars the same as sauerkraut? We've seen a rise in food products with added live microbes, but there haven't been many studies yet. Some studies, though, have suggested that these products contain a much lower number and diversity of microbes.

Probiotic Supplements

In terms of supplements, there's been research but no definitive answers. In the summary study looking at AD, the individual studies used supplements with different types and doses of microbes. Unanswered questions include:

•Can microbes that you eat survive in your gut? For some microbes, the research indicates that they can survive, at least temporarily.

•How can you help these microbes survive? Eat prebiotics. Those good microbes will only thrive if you feed them the right food: fiber-rich prebiotic foods.

•What is the best dose and type of supplement? We definitely need more research: we don't yet know the optimal dose and type.

> **Caution:**
>
> •If you don't have enough good gut microbes, you may have difficulty digesting prebiotic foods.
>
> •The same applies for probiotic foods. Even without gut dysbiosis, some people experience stomach upset and other GI symptoms. If so, introduce these slowly, with a variety of foods to ensure a variety of microbes.

CHAPTER 18
STOP SUGAR SPIKES

Do you really need to read this section if you're in good health, at a normal weight, and feel great? In other words, if your blood sugar levels were elevated, wouldn't you feel it?

Not necessarily.

In fact, there's currently an epidemic of prediabetes and diabetes in the United States, and most of those affected have no symptoms. And this epidemic is affecting plenty of people who don't go near soda or even eat cookies.

You Don't Need To Eat A Lot Of Sugar To Have Elevated Blood Sugar Levels

While consuming too much sugar may play a role, for lots of people it's their OTHER food choices and habits that take a toll. That's the tricky thing about high blood sugar: years of the wrong kind of small habits can add up.

> In recent years, rates of prediabetes and diabetes have risen to shocking levels. These diseases now affect close to 1/3 of Americans (according to a 2015 report from the CDC).
>
> Even more shocking, many don't know it: close to 90% of those with prediabetes don't know it.

That's the case even if your weight is right where it needs to be: there are plenty of people who maintain a normal weight yet still develop elevated blood sugar levels.

Can you be at a normal weight and still have high blood sugar levels? Yes. And your ethnic origin may play a role.

One study looked at Americans with a BMI in the normal range. Of these individuals (who were by definition NOT overweight), African Americans and Hispanics developed metabolic abnormalities at a significantly higher rate than Caucasians. In South Asians, rates were almost twice as high.

Which means that even if you're at a normal weight, you may still be at risk for high fasting blood sugar levels.

And you certainly don't have to have diabetes for your skin to feel the effects of your blood sugar levels. Higher blood sugar levels have been linked to acne and skin inflammation. They've also been linked to aging skin.

The Blood Test You Need at Age 45

You should be tested for prediabetes, even if you have no symptoms and even if you're at a normal weight, when you reach 45. If you're overweight or have other risk factors (such as a relative with diabetes), you should be tested even younger.

Testing involves a simple blood test (you don't even need to fast). This test, called a hemoglobin A1C level, provides an estimate of your blood sugar levels over the previous three months.

Researchers looked at skin aging in over 500 non-diabetic patients.

- They measured glucose levels, and then estimated the age of the volunteers.
- Even after taking into account other factors (including weight, degree of sun damage, and smoking), they discovered that as blood glucose levels increased, perceived age increased.

In other words, higher blood sugar levels make you look older (even if you don't have diabetes).

Strategies to Stop Sugar Spikes

You absolutely have to be careful with the added sugar in your foods and drinks. That slug of sugar-loaded cola is rapidly processed in your digestive system (there's not much to process), and that sugar heads straight to your bloodstream.

But sugary sodas aren't the only cause of elevated blood sugar levels, of course.

To prevent sugar spikes, you need the right strategies. This starts with avoidance of foods heavy in added sugars and refined carbs. It also means focusing on three main strategies: eating the right carbs, eating a half-produce plate, and balancing your carbs with a healthy dose of healthy protein.

Watch Out For Stealth Sugar Bombs
(aka If a Corporation is Adding Sugar to Your Drink, You Need to Know How Much)

I was once at a medical conference, and the physician next to me added 3 teaspoons of sugar to her iced tea. It seemed like a lot.

But then I saw another physician drink down 16 teaspoons of sugar in her coffee.

It's easier than you think. Her Starbucks Caramel Frappucino (medium size) had 16 teaspoons of added sugar.

You'd never add that much yourself, but when somebody else is doing it for you, it's easy to overlook. That's why it's so important to read Nutrition Facts labels, and to check out the websites for your favorite restaurant foods and drinks. You need to know exactly how much sugar Corporation X has shoveled into your food.

Upper Limits for Sugar Consumption

What is considered an OK amount of sugar to consume?

> The American Heart Association recommends (for the average woman) no more than 6 teaspoons of added sugar a day.

There are plenty of stealth sugar bombs that will quickly take you over that limit. Iced Tea. Energy drinks. Coffee drinks. Chai tea lattes.

Even food and drinks with a health halo can be stealth sugar bombs. A carton of Greek yogurt with fruit. Green smoothies. Cold-pressed fresh-squeezed green juice. Even if you're not adding any extra sugar yourself, these foods and beverages may be loaded with added sugar. (One point to emphasize: that upper limit of 6 teaspoons of sugar daily refers to ADDED sugar, not to the sugar that's naturally found in fruit. One other point that's coming up: fruit juice is NOT the same as fruit.)

In fact, it's been estimated that the usual intake of added sugars for Americans is 22 teaspoons per day. That may sound shockingly high (can you imagine sitting there and scooping out 22 teaspoons of sugar from the sugar bowl?). But if you start reading labels, you'll start to see how easy it is to hit that number.

Estimate TSP of Sugar with the Nutrition Facts

> To estimate your sugar intake, take a look at the grams of sugar (listed on the Nutrition Facts). To estimate teaspoons, take the grams of sugar and divide by 4.

If your "lightly sweetened" iced tea has 24 grams of sugar, that's 6 teaspoons of sugar. That's your max for an entire day, right there in just one glass.

Going RIGHT Carb: The Right Type Of Carbs, In The Right Amount, In The Right Company

When it comes to blood sugar, it's not just about the sugar that you eat. Refined carbohydrates have a huge impact on blood sugar levels, which is why choosing the right ones are so important.

Think about the difference between white bread and farro. Although they're both wheat, there's a big difference between the two: one is a highly processed food, and the other is an intact whole grain.

To make white bread, you have to process and pulverize your wheat. In the process, you lose fiber and a number of other nutrients. That's why refined carbs such as white bread and white pasta are sugar spikers: without that fiber, they're quickly digested, which can send blood sugar levels soaring.

Instead, focus on the right type of carbs: power carbs that contain a host of powerful nutrients. These foods naturally contain fiber, along with vitamins, minerals, phytonutrients, and sometimes protein.

Foods that are naturally rich in fiber score better on the glycemic index.

- The glycemic index (GI) is a measure of how much your blood sugar level rises after eating a particular food.
- Foods with a high GI (such as candy bars and white rice) cause sharp, sudden rises in blood sugar levels.
- Foods with a lower GI (such as lentils) are ideal: they lead to a slow, steady rise in blood sugar.
- The glycemic load (GL) is a related measure, which takes into account both the GI of a food (quality) and the portion size (quantity).
- "Mixing" foods can help. For example, adding high-fiber black beans to white rice improves the overall GL

While the fiber in power carbs is important, the other nutrients have important benefits as well. The many vitamins and phytonutrients found in power carbs provide antioxidant and anti-inflammatory benefits, while minerals such as magnesium play a role in regulating blood sugar levels.

Glycemic Load per serving

Higher Glycemic Load (20 or higher): Pancakes, macaroni and cheese, boiled white rice, baked Russet potato, white bagel, fruit leathers, boiled white spaghetti, cornflakes

Intermediate Glycemic Load (11-20): Banana, soda crackers, boiled whole-meal spaghetti, sweet corn on the cob, steamed brown rice, puffed rice cakes

Lower Glycemic Load (10 or lower): Boiled carrots, peanuts, cashews, chickpeas, raw pear, raw orange, raw apple, boiled lentils, boiled kidney beans, whole grain pumpernickel bread, watermelon, 100% whole grain bread

"Mixed Meals": How Beans And Protein Improve The Glycemic Load Of Rice

If white rice has such a high glycemic load, why haven't we historically seen more problems in the Asian countries for which it's a staple food?

The answer is "mixed meals". In Asian countries, white rice is rarely eaten alone. It's usually eaten alongside vegetables, beans, and lentils. Research has shown that eating rice in the company of fiber-rich foods such as beans lowers the glycemic load of the entire meal. The same applies for protein-rich foods: eating carbs alongside protein (such as rice with sushi) lowers the glycemic load of the entire meal. (You still have to keep an eye out for total calories, of course.)

This is an important point to remember as you evaluate the glycemic load of different foods. If you're eating a food by itself (macaroni and cheese), then it may be more of a problem than a food you're eating in company (white rice with black beans).

Everybody's Different: Variability in GL Responses

Another important point about GL values: they only provide a relative estimate of a food's effects on blood sugar levels. Because there's such a wide variability in individual blood sugar responses to foods, you should evaluate any published glycemic load values as only relative estimates.

The Right Amount: You Still Need To Watch Portion Sizes, Even With The Right Carbs

I talk about choosing the right type of carbs more than I talk about going "low carb", because there's a big difference between a piece of white bread and a bowl of lentil soup.

However, many of us should be lowering our overall carb intake. Many Americans are eating too many refined, processed carbs, and eating less of these foods is an easy health strategy. But even if all you're eating are power carbs, you still need to watch your portion sizes. The fiber and protein in these are great for your blood sugar, but they can only do so much; eat enough brown rice, and you CAN send your blood sugar soaring.

It's also important to recognize that we all have different responses to the same quantity of carbohydrates. Some individuals seem to be more sensitive to carbs, with even a reasonable amount sending their blood sugar levels soaring. Later in this section you'll read more about carbohydrate sensitivity.

The Half-Produce Plate Ensures That You Fill Up On Fiber

The Healthy Eating Plate (created by the USDA and available at www.ChooseMyPlate.gov), and the modified, more detailed version known as the Harvard Healthy Eating Plate, provide a great strategy to keep blood sugar levels stable. It's a great way to eyeball your plate and know if you're on track.

Half of your plate should be covered in vegetables and fruit (with more vegetables than fruit), while about ¼ should be a serving of healthy carbohydrates and about ¼ should be a serving of healthy protein. I call this the half-produce plate.

When half of your dinner plate is covered by mainly vegetables, you're consuming a hefty dose of powerful nutrients, and especially a hefty dose of fiber.

You Need A Nice Dose Of Healthy Protein On Your Plate To Balance Out Your Carbs: Balanced Meals Mean Steady Blood Sugars

Although it might have been your favorite meal in college, a bowl of cereal for dinner is a definite sugar spiker. Without any protein or fat to slow them down, those carbs are quickly released into the bloodstream.

No more cereal for dinner. Your carbs need a healthy dose of healthy protein to balance them out.

If you think back to the healthy plate, about ¼ of your plate should be a healthy protein source.

That protein provides the building blocks for muscle, hair, and skin. It also acts to stabilize blood sugar levels. A reasonable serving of fat helps too: it helps stabilize blood sugar levels and it's required for the absorption of certain vitamins.

It's Not Just About The Macronutrients: Micronutrients Also Matter

While we know all about the importance of the right kind of carbs, it turns out that micronutrients are also important when it comes to stabilizing blood sugar levels. Minerals such as magnesium (found in many whole foods, including beans, nuts, and seeds) and chromium have been shown to play a role in keeping blood glucose and insulin levels stable. Spices may also play a role: some of the phytonutrients found in spices such as cinnamon and fenugreek are being studied for their potential role in helping to stabilize blood sugar levels.

Personalized Nutrition: Why Some of Us May Need to Watch Our Carb Intake

There's a common question debated on health blogs, and I'm sure you've heard it. **Are carbs good or bad for you?**

In response, I would ask: What do you mean by carbs? **And who are you?**

The first part of that question was discussed in the section on power carbs. Carbs are not created equal, and you really need to focus on the right type of carbs.

But the second part of that question is equally important. Although we don't yet know all of the factors that play into this, research has found that some people do seem to be more sensitive to carbohydrates.

We all need to eat a combination of protein, carbs, and fat: those are the three macronutrients. We all consume these in different proportions, and there's a range that's considered fine for most active individuals. The Food and Nutrition Board of the Institutes of Medicine states that an acceptable range is:

- Carbohydrates 45-65% of energy
- Protein 10-35% of energy
- Fat 20-35% of energy

That's the range, but what's the ideal number? Based on all the research that's been done to date, there doesn't seem to be an ideal ratio that works for every single person. However, there does appear to be a better ratio that works for individuals. That's because people can have widely different responses to the identical amount of carbohydrates.

Some People Seem To Be More Sensitive To Carbs

Some people can eat a banana, and their blood sugar barely budges. Another person, eating that same banana, will see her blood sugar shoot up. We know that this happens, but we don't yet understand all of the factors that determine your body's response to carbohydrates.

In one study, researchers asked 800 volunteers to wear a continuous glucose monitoring device. Then they fed them identical meals and measured their blood sugar levels.

There were startling differences. Some people had very high sugar spikes after the meal, while blood sugar levels barely budged in others.

Why would some people be that much more sensitive to eating carbs? We don't know for sure. Researchers looked at the data, and they found multiple factors that seemed to be associated with carb sensitivity.

- These factors included a person's age.
- It also included their weight.
- It also included their medical conditions, such as blood pressure.
- It also included overall levels of inflammation in their body, as measured by C-reactive protein blood levels.
- It even included the composition of their gut bacteria.

While we don't yet understand all of the factors that determine carb sensitivity, it's clear that some people may be highly sensitive to carbs. For these individuals, it may be helpful to carefully monitor and limit portion sizes.

It's also important to emphasize that our sensitivity to carbs changes as we get older. Some people become more sensitive to carbohydrates with age. This is an important point, because it means that what worked for you in your 20s (cereal for breakfast) may not work for you in your 30s.

Determining Your Own Response To Carbs

It can be tricky to figure out if you're carb sensitive. One of the important research studies in this area made use of a continuous blood glucose monitor, which provides a steady stream of blood sugar readings. Even without technology though, you can still start with a food diary and some experimentation. A nutritionist and your physician may also be able to provide some guidelines.

The Mid-Morning Energy Slump

Here's how I figured out I was carb sensitive: my response to breakfast. For years, I had cereal for breakfast every single morning. (And I never skipped breakfast, because it's the most important meal of the day.) One year I noticed that I couldn't get through my morning clinic without having to take a break. Around 11AM, I'd be starving and starting to lose my concentration, and I'd need a banana to fix things quickly.

Everything changed when I started eating breakfast tacos. Breakfast tacos are simple: eggs scrambled with vegetables, wrapped up in a whole wheat tortilla, with a sprinkling of shredded cheese. With my egg for breakfast, I stayed full until 1pm, and my mind stayed sharp. (And I lost 12 pounds.)

Protein For Breakfast
Stabilized My Blood Sugar Levels

The medical explanation is that my blood sugar levels were finally stable all morning.

One of the major tenets of eating for younger skin is "stop sugar spikes." Those sugar spikes impact your entire body, often causing silent damage. But sometimes you <u>will</u> feel the symptoms of sugar spikes, due to the rollercoaster effect.

The Rollercoaster Effect:
Sugar Spikes Followed By Sugar Crashes

When you have a giant bowl of breakfast cereal, heavy on the carbs and without any protein to balance it, your blood sugar levels may shoot up. That causes your insulin levels to shoot up in response.

Insulin is the hormone that jumps in and moves that sugar out of your bloodstream and into your cells. But when insulin has to work so quickly and at such high levels, it can sometimes overshoot the mark. Sometimes it clears out too much blood sugar, which results in plunging levels of blood sugar.

In other words, you're left with a sugar crash. That's the rollercoaster effect: high blood sugar levels (for some people) are followed by low blood sugar levels.

You know what low blood sugar levels feel like. They're why you get "hangry": you're starving and you're irritable and you can't focus. (Which is the scientific explanation for why it's so hard to pick a restaurant when you're starving.) These are all signs that your brain is feeling the effects of low blood sugar.

Should You Go Low Carb?

For most Americans, it's safe to say that we're probably eating too many carbs right now, and cutting carbs is a quick and easy way to achieve health benefits and lose weight. But while cutting carbs may help, you don't have to go truly low carb to see benefits on your skin.

If you're truly going low carb, you're getting less than 45% of your calories from sources of carbohydrates. If you're on a medical ketogenic diet, you're going lower than that. These diets may be recommended for certain medical conditions, but they should be done with medical supervision.

In terms of your skin, just going right carb can help.

Right Carb Diets (Right Type of Carbs, Right Amount) May Help Some People With Acne

- In one experiment, patients with acne were asked to follow a low glycemic load diet for 12 weeks.
- They were asked to choose the right types of carbs, and they were asked to replace some of their carbs with protein.
- This was NOT a low carb diet and it was NOT a low fat diet: these volunteers were asked to get 25% of energy from protein/ 45% from low GI carbs/ and 30% from fat. This falls right into the range of recommended proportions.
- After 12 weeks, the volunteers had a notable improvement in their acne.
- They also had lower levels of acne-worsening hormone levels.
- Later studies using skin biopsies even showed less skin inflammation.
- This approach does not work for all patients with acne, since there are multiple other factors that impact acne.

OTHER STRATEGIES

Salad (With Vinegar) First, Bread Last

When the waiter offers you a salad before your meal, opt in and order a vinaigrette dressing. Research has shown that vinegar at the start of a meal acts to blunt sugar levels after a meal.

In other words, that salad with vinegar can help reduce sugar spikes.

The bread basket, on the other hand, gets saved for later. In one small study, people with diabetes had a 30% higher blood sugar level when they started their meal with bread, as opposed to ending their meal with bread. That's enough to recommend holding off on the bread basket until AFTER you've gotten some protein into your system.

Think Fruit, Not Juice

This is how the theory goes: since there are so many great phytonutrients in fruit, wouldn't juice provide those phytonutrients in a powerful, concentrated form?

While it sounds good in theory, fruit juices just aren't the same as fruit. Studies suggest that when you take nutrients out of their fiber matrix, your body responds to them differently. When you're juicing, you're discarding the pulp. But that pulp is fiber, and fiber is important. In fact, while consuming whole fruit on a regular basis may reduce your risk of diabetes, drinking juice on a regular basis actually INCREASES your risk.

One study looked at the effects of fruit versus fruit juice. Fruit was WAY better.

People who ate whole fruits such as berries, grapes, and apples (at least twice a week) cut their risk of diabetes by 23% (as opposed to those who ate fruit just once a month).

For fruit juice, it was the exact opposite. Those who drank a serving or more every day INCREASED their risk by up to 21%.

High Protein Breakfast

A lot of us grew up eating cereal for breakfast. But as you get older, your ability to process carbohydrates may not be as strong. (I know that was the case for me when I hit my 30s).

That's one of the reasons why a high-protein breakfast may be a good strategy to reduce sugar spikes. For many people, the highest blood sugars that they'll experience tend to be after breakfast. This may be because stress hormones such as cortisol are increased in your bloodstream during the early morning. That makes your body more insulin resistant, which means your insulin doesn't work as well, which means your blood sugar levels may start to spike. High protein breakfasts help limit those blood sugar spikes.

Spice Up Your Meals

Add cinnamon to your oatmeal and turmeric with sautéed onions to your scrambled eggs. You'll be adding more than just flavor: research suggests that spices may help reduce blood sugar levels and improve insulin resistance. While experts aren't such of the exact mechanism of action, or the doses required to achieve these effects, we know from centuries of use that adding spices to your food is safe.

Spices that have been shown in research studies to improve blood sugar levels include (and there are more) cinnamon, cloves, black cumin seeds, coriander seeds, fennel, fenugreek, ginger, and turmeric. Onions aren't a spice, but they're a great way to spice up your food, and they've also shown benefits.

Go Nuts

Adding some nuts to your salad is a simple and effective strategy, since their healthy fats and fiber help keep blood sugar levels stable. They're also a source of minerals (such as magnesium) that may be helpful in blood sugar regulation. Since they're a concentrated source of calories, though, you'll need to watch out for portion sizes.

> Patients with diabetes who snacked on 1 ounce of pistachios twice a day experienced lower hemoglobin A-1 C levels and lower levels of inflammation (as measured by C-reactive protein levels).

Take A Walk After Dinner

What you eat at the dinner table is important. But what you do after you get up can also have a big   impact.

In many countries, families get up from the dinner table and then go for an after-dinner stroll. (As opposed to the other after-dinner tradition: flop on the couch and turn on the TV.)

Researchers found that a 10-minute walk after meals had definite benefits.

In this study, a group of volunteers was instructed to eat breakfast or lunch or dinner, and then, within five minutes, head out for a brief 10-minute walk. This one strategy resulted in post-meal blood sugar levels that were 12% lower overall.

Take A (Brief) Walk During Work

Taking short (just 2 minutes long) walks throughout your workday may not sound like much, but research has shown that those short walks may improve your blood sugar levels. In one experiment, researchers compared blood glucose levels in volunteers who stayed sitting during their day, versus those who got up every 20 minutes and took a light-intensity 2-minute walk. That one simple change resulted in better overall blood glucose levels following a sugary drink.

CHAPTER 19
STOP SKIN SABOTAGE

If Sunday brunch with your friends is a weekly tradition, then the choices you make with your fork every week can add up to a hearty dose of skin saving nutrients.

Or a hefty dose of skin damage.

In the preceding section, you learned all about strategies to maintain stable blood sugar levels. The whole goal of those guidelines is to avoid excess blood sugar, which triggers the formation of sugar protein complexes. Those compounds, known as AGEs, are known collagen threats.

Sugar isn't the only threat to your skin though. Some foods, such as that bacon you love with brunch, come loaded with their own pre-formed AGEs. And research has found that the AGEs you eat are absorbed into your bloodstream and go on to cause the same kind of damage.

> In a study looking at the level of AGEs found in different foods, bacon was one of the top offenders.

AGEs In Food: What To Look Out For

- Vegetables, beverages, and carbohydrates have lower levels of pre-formed AGEs
- Meats have higher levels
- Cooking methods make a big difference in the levels of AGEs
- In general, browning of food is a sign of glycation
- Cooking with dry heat, such as by roasting or broiling, dramatically raises levels of AGEs
- Cooking with fat raises them even more, such as pan-frying or deep-frying
- For cooking methods that don't raise levels of AGEs much, try cooking with moist heat, such as steaming or poaching
- Although roasting and grilling vegetables raises the level of AGEs, the final amount is still much, much lower than what you'd find in meat
- The processing methods used on some foods can also increase the AGE count, such as with whipped butter
- Crackers, chips, and cookies are other concerning sources of AGEs, likely due to dry-heat processing and ingredients such as butter, oil, and cheese

For a general idea of the AGEs found in different foods, see the list below.

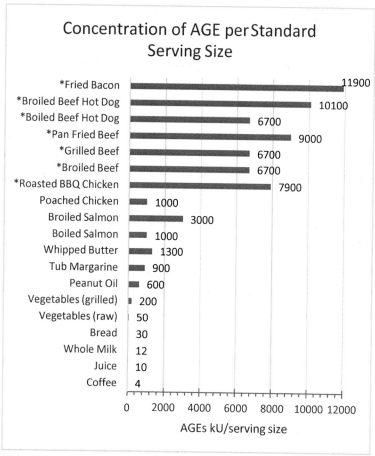

Concentration of AGE per Standard Serving Size

Food	AGEs kU/serving size
*Fried Bacon	11900
*Broiled Beef Hot Dog	10100
*Boiled Beef Hot Dog	6700
*Pan Fried Beef	9000
*Grilled Beef	6700
*Broiled Beef	6700
*Roasted BBQ Chicken	7900
Poached Chicken	1000
Broiled Salmon	3000
Boiled Salmon	1000
Whipped Butter	1300
Tub Margarine	900
Peanut Oil	600
Vegetables (grilled)	200
Vegetables (raw)	50
Bread	30
Whole Milk	12
Juice	10
Coffee	4

AGEs kU/serving size

*Adapted from data in/ reprinted with permission from *Journal of the American Dietetic Association*, Volume 110/Edition 6, Uribarri J, Woodruff S, Goodman S, et al, Advanced Glycation End Products in Foods and a Practical Guide to Their Reduction in the Diet, 911-16, Copyright 2010, with permission from Elsevier and American Dietetic Association.

Trans Fats Accelerate Skin Aging

What happens if you were to eat your favorite packaged cookies, 3 every day, for months at a time? (And by packaged cookies, I'm talking about the type that could live in the back of your pantry for 2 years and would still be crispy and tasty when you finally found them.) In terms of your skin, that daily dose of packaged cookies could be accelerating the skin aging process.

That's because of trans fats. If there's one food villain just about everybody agrees on, it's trans fats. These are substances that were created in a laboratory. They were initially celebrated, because adding trans fats to processed foods means that those foods can live on a shelf much longer. But those trans fats do more than just make cookies last longer-they've been shown to increase the risk of several diseases, including heart disease.

They're also bad for your skin.

In one study, lab animals were fed a hydrogenated vegetable oil heavy in trans fats. They were then exposed to UV radiation for 12 weeks. At the end of that time, they produced more free radicals and fewer skin antioxidants.

Trans fats are so harmful that they'll be banned in the United States starting in 2018. Common sources include:

- Processed foods that list trans fats on the Nutrition Facts labels
- Processed foods that list 0 grams of trans fats on the Nutrition Facts, but still list partially hydrogenated oils in the ingredient list. This is due to a loophole in the labeling laws: if a food contains less than 0.5 grams per serving of trans fats, it may legally state 0 grams of trans fats on the Nutrition Facts label
- Foods fried in partially hydrogenated oils, such as in some restaurants. (Have you ever asked your favorite fast food restaurant/ casual dining restaurant/ fine dining restaurant what kind of oil they use for your favorite French fries?)

Section 3

DIET AND DERMATOLOGY

The focus of this book has been on dietary recommendations for maintaining youthful skin.

The same recommendations form the foundation of eating for acne, eczema, psoriasis, and rosacea.

That's because each of these skin conditions involves inflammation of the skin, and a diet based on whole foods serves as the foundation for an anti-inflammatory diet. The focus on foods that are rich in fiber and that help maintain a healthy gut is also helpful for some of these skin conditions. Studies on eczema have found that a combination of pre-biotics and probiotics may help in treatment of the skin symptoms, while research in rosacea patients has found a higher risk of GI conditions such as irritable bowel syndrome.

The following section has a brief summary of the diet recommendations for each of these skin conditions, broken down into potential trigger foods and helper foods. For a more extensive discussion, please see my website www.SkinAndDiet.com. You'll find links there to several of my articles (written for a medical audience) that go into much more detail. Since research is ongoing, I maintain a blog with regular updates. There's still so much that we don't know, which is why we so strongly advocate for more research into chronic skin diseases.

One very important point: changing your diet is only one aspect of dealing with a chronic skin condition. Despite what you may have seen on the Internet, there is no special diet or special supplement that's been proven to cure psoriasis. However, eating a nutrient-rich diet that focuses on whole foods as opposed to processed foods can, in some cases, help your treatment be more effective.

Summary of Skin Conditions and Food Triggers

*Children are at higher risk for nutritional deficiencies. Always speak to your pediatrician before eliminating foods

Skin Condition	Potential food triggers	Recommended tests
Acne	• Sugar and refined carbohydrates • Role of dairy and whey protein varies	• 12-week diet change
Aging Skin	• Sugar, refined carbohydrates • Fried foods • Meats grilled at high temperatures • Trans fats	
Eczema/ atopic dermatitis	Type 1 Hypersensitivity Reactions: Eggs, milk, wheat, soy, seafood, and nuts	• Skin prick tests or blood tests • Confirm with physician-supervised food challenge
	Delayed eczematous reactions: Eggs, milk, wheat, soy, seafood, and nuts	• Food diary • Confirm with physician-supervised food challenge
	Systemic contact dermatitis: Foods related to balsam of Peru, foods high in nickel, processed foods containing propylene glycol	• Food diary • Confirm with patch testing

Skin Condition	Potential food triggers	Recommended Tests
Rosacea	• Alcohol • Heat related: coffee, tea • Capsaicin-related: peppers, spicy foods • Cinnamaldehyde-related: tomatoes, citrus, chocolate, cinnamon	• Food diary • 6-week avoidance diet
Psoriasis	• Pro-inflammatory foods (sugar, refined carbs, unhealthy fats) may increase risk of associated systemic diseases	
	• Gluten may act as a food trigger in a small percentage of psoriasis patients	• Blood tests for gluten antibodies • Evaluation by GI doctor for those with symptoms

*As in other areas, everyone is different, and the research in these areas is evolving. Your dermatologic and medical history will always impact dietary recommendations

CHAPTER 20
ACNE

SUCCESS REPORTED When it comes to acne, there are multiple factors at play, including genetics and hormones. For some people, their diet is another factor. Based on experiments, some people with acne have improved when they switched to eating a low glycemic load diet.

While dermatologists (for decades) doubted a relationship between diet and acne, that's now changed. A thorough review in 2010 by Drs. Bowe, Joshi, and Shalita revisited the earlier research, and found flaws in some of the earlier studies. More recent research has provided stronger evidence, including randomized controlled trials (RCTs). This type of research involves an experiment, and it's considered one of the best types of evidence for proving a link between diet and health.

> In one experiment (by Dr. Smith and colleagues in Melbourne), researchers worked with a group of male patients who all had acne. They randomly assigned the patients to two groups.
>
> One group ate a low glycemic load (GL) diet for 12 weeks. The other group ate their regular diet.
>
> At the end of 12 weeks, the patients on a low GL diet experienced significantly more improvement in their acne.

In this study, one group was asked to follow a low glycemic load (low GL) diet. A low GL diet takes into account the quantity of carbohydrates consumed, as well as quality, by focusing on foods with a lower glycemic index. The glycemic index (GI) is a measure of how much your blood sugar level rises after eating a particular food.

As an example of diet changes in this study, volunteers ate whole grain bread instead of white bread. They also reduced their total carbohydrate intake by replacing high GI foods with foods that were higher in protein, such as fish and poultry.

This was not a low carb diet, since carbs made up 45% of the diet. Instead, it focused on the quality and quantity of carbs.

QUALITY: Whole grain bread instead of white

QUANTITY: Cut out high GI foods and replace them with higher protein foods

It's important to realize that they were NOT asked to follow a low carb diet. Their recommended diet plan was designed to provide 25% of energy from protein/ 45% from low GI carbs/ and 30% from fat. The suggested diet was also designed to provide the same number of calories as their previous diet.

The other group of volunteers served as a comparison group. They were asked to eat foods that were similar to their regular diet, with carbs that had moderate to high GI values.

Both groups followed their diet plan for 12 weeks, and the results were clear. The volunteers in the low GL group had fewer red bumps and pustules. They even had fewer whiteheads and blackheads.

Other research studies have found similar results. Testing has even shown that a low GL diet causes beneficial changes in hormone levels and skin sebum production. Skin biopsies of volunteers after a low GL diet have found smaller sebaceous (oil) glands and less skin inflammation.

Of course, it's important to realize that diet is only one possible factor in acne. The largest causes still remain genetics and hormonal changes, especially those related to puberty. It's also important to recognize that even if the skin improves, many patients will still require medicated acne treatments.

TRIGGERS Added sugars and refined carbohydrates can worsen acne in some people, because they act to spike blood sugar levels. This can increase the levels of certain hormones that promote skin inflammation.

The issue of dairy and acne is still unclear. We definitely need more research, but it does seem as though some people (not all) are more sensitive to dairy when it comes to acne. In one report, five teenagers developed treatment-resistant acne after starting whey protein supplements. (Whey comes from dairy.)

HELPERS In terms of foods that might help in acne, studies in humans are limited. Foods that are naturally rich in fiber are suggested, especially because they stabilize blood sugar levels. There has been some interesting research that suggests that omega-3 fatty acids and probiotics may help. There's also been interesting research into zinc, a mineral with anti-inflammatory properties. Although more research is needed, foods such as red kidney beans and shrimp are good sources of zinc.

CHAPTER 21
ECZEMA

SUCCESS REPORTED Atopic dermatitis, commonly known as eczema, can be a very frustrating skin condition. There are multiple factors that play a role in causing skin flares, and there's still so much that we don't yet understand about how these all work together. Sometimes, even if you're doing everything right, your skin can still flare. Having said that, working to maximize every factor that's under your control is still important.

> One summary study looked at the results of experiments that tested synbiotics for the treatment of eczema.
>
> Overall, the use of synbiotics (combinations of prebiotics and probiotics) for at least 8 weeks in adults and children over the age of 1 year old had a significant effect on eczema severity.

TRIGGERS The issue of food allergies in eczema is very complex. We know that patients with atopic dermatitis experience food allergies at a higher rate than others. In some cases, although not all, these food allergies may trigger a flare of atopic dermatitis.

A food diary may help identify some possible food allergies. Testing is then needed for confirmation. In children, we never recommend eliminating foods until testing is done, because of the risk of nutritional deficiencies.

Testing for food allergies is actually a very complex area: please see my website for more details on the limitations of food allergy testing.

> There are at least 3 different types of food allergies (and possibly more) that can act to trigger flares of eczema, and each requires a different approach.

Some food allergies (known as IgE-mediated) result in reactions within minutes to hours. The top triggers are milk, eggs, wheat, soy, nuts, and seafood. Delayed eczematous reactions result in flares of eczema up to 2 days later, and the top trigger foods are the same. Systemic contact dermatitis can also result in a delayed flare of eczema. One of the top triggers is in persons allergic to fragrance additives in their skin care products. Related foods can trigger a rash, and these include cinnamon, tomatoes, citrus, and chocolate.

HELPERS In terms of foods that may help in the treatment of atopic dermatitis, the most promise has been seen with synbiotics. Synbiotics are probiotics in combination with prebiotics. Research studies have looked at the results of synbiotics when used in conjunction with standard eczema treatments.

In one summary paper, researchers found that the most promise in the treatment of atopic dermatitis was seen with probiotics that used multiple strains of bacteria, in combination with prebiotics, when given for at least 8 weeks to adults and children over the age of 1. There's much more research necessary, though, before we can be sure of what to recommend. We still don't know what types of probiotics would be best, especially in terms of bacterial strains, dosage, and formulation.

We can certainly recommend eating for a healthy gut with the use of prebiotic and probiotic foods.

> Maintaining a healthy gut ensures the growth of good microbes. These microbes are able to produce short chain fatty acids. SCFAs are substances that may help strengthen the skin barrier. Some power fats, such as omega-3 fatty acids, have also shown promise in reducing skin irritation and moisture loss.

Vitamin D has been studied for its possible role in the treatment of eczema, but more research is needed. Preliminary research suggests that it may be helpful in those with very low levels of vitamin D, those who have food allergies, and those who experience frequent bacterial skin infections.

CHAPTER 22
PSORIASIS

SUCCESS REPORTED A healthy anti-inflammatory diet is very important for patients with psoriasis. That's because patients with psoriasis have a higher risk of high blood pressure, diabetes, and heart disease. The good news is that the right eating patterns can help reduce those risks.

In terms of treating the skin findings of psoriasis, the dietary research is not as complete. There have been several studies showing that a diet and exercise program that leads to weight loss in those who are overweight has resulted in improved response to certain psoriasis treatments. These programs have also led to improved skin symptoms, with an improved PASI score (Psoriasis Area and Severity Index) in some (not all) patients. More research is needed to see if anti-inflammatory eating patterns can improve the skin findings of psoriasis.

> Diet and exercise programs leading to weight loss may improve psoriasis severity.
>
> A summary report of five such programs in overweight psoriasis patients found that patients who lost weight on the programs experienced an overall improvement in psoriasis severity scores.

TRIGGERS In terms of triggers, the biggest lifestyle factors that may worsen psoriasis in some patients are smoking and increased alcohol intake.

Gluten-containing foods may act as a trigger in some patients, but it's not a common trigger. For patients with GI symptoms (such as constipation/diarrhea/abdominal pain/ other symptoms), we recommend testing for celiac antibodies. Several studies have found that patients with psoriasis are at about double the risk for developing celiac disease. That's still not a high number, though, since celiac disease is so uncommon in most populations. Other patients with psoriasis don't have celiac disease, but do have certain gluten antibodies. Some of these patients have noticed improvement by avoiding gluten. Blood tests can identify these antibodies.

HELPERS The research suggests that for overweight psoriasis patients, diet and exercise programs leading to weight loss may help. However, we still need more research into whether a particular type of diet may help. In terms of supplements, we need more research, especially into fish oil and vitamin D. Curcumin, the active ingredient in the spice turmeric, also warrants more research.

CHAPTER 23
ROSACEA

SUCCESS REPORTED If you have rosacea, it's possible that eliminating certain "trigger" foods may help. In one survey of patients by the National Rosacea Society, 78% had altered their diet, and 95% of this group reported fewer flares afterwards. The triggers seemed to fall into 4 main groups.

- Alcohol
- Hot beverages, such as coffee and tea
- Capsaicin-related, including spices and hot sauce
- Cinnamaldehyde-related (tomatoes/chocolate/citrus)

TRIGGERS We definitely need more research into dietary triggers. Since surveys suggest they play a role, I recommend keeping a food diary. Another option is 6 weeks avoidance of the common triggers. If you experience improvement, you can then reintroduce each food, one at a time, every few days, to see if you can pinpoint your particular triggers.

HELPERS More research is needed, but there does seem to be a gut-skin connection in rosacea.

One study of close to 50,000 patients with rosacea found that they had a higher prevalence of certain GI conditions (including celiac disease, small intestinal bacterial overgrowth, and irritable bowel syndrome).

Given this finding, foods that maintain good gut health may be important, including foods that are naturally rich in fiber and foods that contain probiotics.

CHAPTER 24
MORE RESEARCH NEEDED

The intersection of diet and skin conditions is an area where we're seeing a lot more research studies. These are just some of the areas I've written about and which I'm following closely for new developments:

1. FOOD ALLERGIES

The incidence of food allergies has risen dramatically over the last 20 years. There also seems to be a rise in food sensitivities and food intolerances.

There are lots of theories about why the incidence of food allergies and food sensitivities has been rising, but we don't have definite answers. That means that this area is prone to unproven or false information, and you need to be cautious with what you read.

> Food allergy is a surprisingly complex area. There are different types of food allergies, and different types of tests required. In some cases of food allergies, we just don't know the exact immune system pathway that's involved.
>
> That means that we don't have a single easy blood test or skin test that covers all types of food allergies.

There's also the issue of food sensitivities and food intolerances, where symptoms occur after eating a food but we haven't been able to trace the symptoms back to a particular immune system pathway. I've spoken to patients who report that certain foods seem to trigger GI symptoms, skin symptoms, and even joint symptoms. While some have improved with avoiding the suspected food, their symptoms don't follow the pattern of typical food allergy. That's why these symptoms are termed food "sensitivity" or "intolerance".

Until we know more, I keep an open mind along with a great deal of caution. Elimination diets do carry their own risks (loss of nutrients, substitution with less healthy foods), so I recommend starting with a food diary. Some clinics will perform blinded food challenges, in which the suspect food or a placebo is given to the patient, followed by monitoring for symptoms. While there are other types of food testing available, for some we just don't have good data yet on the rates of false negative and false positive tests. Research is ongoing as to the best tests for these different food reactions. Which brings me to my next area of interest:

2. THE GUT-SKIN CONNECTION

I've noticed over the last few years that more of my dermatology patients are describing irritable bowel syndrome or other GI conditions as a part of their medical history. I've certainly had more patients than ever asking if there's a link between their diet and their skin.

This is an area that definitely needs more research.

In eczema, several studies have found some benefits with synbiotics (used alongside proven treatments). Synbiotics combine prebiotics and probiotics. Prebiotics are foods that support the growth of "good" gut microbes, while probiotics are foods or supplements that contain good microbes.

Many research studies have shown that these "good" germs have an important role to play in our GI tract. They're critical for our gut health, because they digest the fiber in our food and extract important nutrients. They also protect us from bad microbes, protect the lining of our gut, help train the immune system, and produce beneficial, anti-inflammatory substances called short chain fatty acids (SCFAs). These SCFAs act to enhance and protect our gut lining and our skin barrier.

More clues to a gut-skin link have been found in other skin conditions. For example, in a study of over 50,000 patients with rosacea, it was found that rosacea patients had a higher prevalence of many different types of GI disorders, including irritable bowel syndrome and small intestinal bacterial overgrowth.

This link is important, because studies suggest rising rates of irritable bowel syndrome in this country. While there are many unanswered questions and potential causes, one of the theories centers on gut dysbiosis. In gut dysbiosis, there's an imbalance of good microbes and bad microbes. While nobody knows for sure why gut dysbiosis seems to be rising, one theory is that the use of antibacterial products and antibiotics are killing off our good microbes. Another reason is the typical American diet. A diet that's lower in fiber and higher in sugar and refined carbohydrates promotes the loss of good gut microbes.

That loss of good microbes may partially explain certain GI symptoms. If you don't have enough good gut microbes, then you may have difficulty digesting certain foods. This may help explain why gluten-free diets and low FODMAP diets help some patients with gut dysbiosis.

Some researchers have suggested that a loss of good gut microbes may partially explain the development of some food hypersensitivities. Patients with gut dysbiosis may develop a loss of the tight barrier function of the innermost lining of the gut. (In medical terms, increased intestinal permeability.) That means that the immune cells located in the wall of your gut may have more exposure to food. With more exposure, you may be more likely to develop food allergies or hypersensitivities. We don't yet have proof of these theories, but research is ongoing.

3. MICRONUTRIENTS

The micronutrients in foods (including vitamins and minerals) are essential for good health. They're also essential for healthy skin: deficiencies can lead to poor wound healing (vitamin C) to hair loss (iron and zinc) to inflamed tongues (vitamin B12) to many others.

And in today's world, with the rise of heavily processed foods and industrialized food systems, we're starting to worry about these even more. We're seeing scurvy (vitamin C deficiency) in people who subsist on processed foods, and we're starting to worry about food that's grown in overfarmed, poor soil.

That's already been shown to be a problem in some parts of the world. For example, selenium deficiency is seen in some places because the soil doesn't contain enough of this important mineral. Magnesium deficiency in our soil and foods is also a concern, especially since magnesium is important in blood sugar control.

Creating highly processed foods also results in fewer micronutrients. We may not know what we're missing out on until later, when symptoms of nutrient deficiencies start to appear.

> Some experts believe that the rise of vampires in Europe was due to processed food. (Really.)

When corn spread from America to Europe, and cornmeal became a staple food among the poor, symptoms of niacin deficiency became widespread. That's because while the traditional processing methods used in the Americas ensured the bioavailability of niacin, those practices were not adopted in Europe. Niacin deficiency results in pellagra, and it's been suggested that widespread pellagra may have led to the myths of vampires. Pellagra results in extreme sun sensitivity, "bloody" gums (inflamed gums and tongue), and eventual dementia.

We certainly need more research on what types of deficiencies we may be at risk for. We also need more research on the best laboratory testing to identify deficiencies of micronutrients. Some of these micronutrients are stored in our organs, and blood tests may not be the most accurate measure of their levels.

4. ARE THERE OTHER, YET-TO-BE-RECOGNIZED EFFECTS OF PROCESSED FOODS?

Apart from micronutrients, what other effects of processed foods do we need to be on the lookout for? One concern is that with more processed foods, it's possible that our bodies may use fewer calories when digesting and processing those foods.

"Metabolic energy expenditure" refers to how many calories we use over the course of a day. Most of our calorie usage is related to our basal metabolic rate (how many calories we use to keep the body functioning at rest) and our active metabolic rate (calories used during physical activity). But some of our calories are used in the process of breaking down our food, making enzymes, absorbing nutrients, and other related functions. This is known as postprandial (after meals) energy expenditure, and it's thought to account for about 10% of our daily calorie usage.

One study compared calories used by the body after a whole foods (WF) meal versus a processed food (PF) meal. (These contained equivalent protein/carbs/fat.) One example used multi-grain bread with cheddar cheese versus white bread with processed cheese.

There was a notable difference in calories used: the PF meal expended only about half of the calories of the WF meal. With these concerning initial results, more research in this area is recommended.

5. IS THERE A PROBLEM WITH PULVERIZING?

One of the areas I'm following closely is the effect of pulverizing our food. In other words, what happens when you smash a food into tiny particles? Does your body still react to it in the same way? Protein, fiber, and power carbs are important skin nutrients, and they're being processed in this way more frequently.

Take quinoa pasta or whole wheat bread. If you start with a whole grain, then pulverize it thoroughly, and then reshape it, does it change your body's response to that food? Would you experience different effects in the digestive system and on blood glucose levels from such a food as compared to an intact whole grain such as farro?

I have the same questions about pea protein. What happens when you take peas, pulverize them, and then add them back to granola bars in the form of pea protein? Does that pea protein function in the body the same way that it would if you ate actual peas?

It's clear we need more research on these questions, especially as more and more processed foods are relying on techniques or additives such as these to try to improve their health profile.

CHAPTER 25

WHEN HEALTH MARKETING JUST DOESN'T TELL THE FULL STORY

I've seen a lot of ideas floating around the internet on how to achieve healthy skin. You need to be aware that some of the promised "quick-fixes" out there just don't tell the full story.

1. Nutritional supplements. Please, please be careful when deciding whether or not to take a particular supplement. Just because they're touted as "natural" doesn't necessarily mean that they're safe or effective. First, supplements aren't regulated the way that medications are. (Legally, supplements are regulated as foods, not drugs.) Manufacturers of supplements don't have to prove that they're effective or that they're safe before they start selling them. Sometimes there's a lack of quality control: some supplements have been found to be mixed with toxic metals (lead, mercury) while others have contained potent pharmaceutical ingredients, like steroids. Others don't contain the advertised dose of ingredients.

Even if the supplement contains high-quality ingredients at the dose specified, it may not be the right supplement for you. I've seen many hair loss supplements that contain vitamin A, even though at high doses this vitamin can actually cause hair loss. **The bottom line: With all supplements, make sure you're taking the right supplement at the right dose for the right condition.**

2. Herbal products. Whether it's labeled a "nutritional supplement" or an "herbal product", the same rule applies. Whether it's Chinese herbs, Ayurvedic herbs, or herbal supplements sold at your drugstore, you have to do your homework. Some herbs have evidence supporting their use, but you can't just rely on a single term on the label. Exactly what is in this product? Is it safe for your medical profile? Is it the right product and the right dose for you? Was it tested for contamination? Even if it's the exact product indicated, many herbs have the potential for side effects or medication interactions. Bottom line: do your homework instead of just relying on the term "herbal" on the label.

3. Probiotics: Taking a probiotic supplement and stopping there isn't as important as eating well. The live microbes in probiotic foods, and sometimes supplements, can help promote a healthy gut, which can help your skin and overall health. But probiotics by themselves aren't enough: they should always be used with prebiotic foods. In other words, you can eat "good microbes", but if those microbes are going to successfully live and thrive in your gut, they're going to need the right type of food. And that means fiber.

3. "High-fiber" processed foods. Speaking of fiber, we just don't know if the fiber added to processed foods functions the same way in the body as the fiber in vegetables. Manufacturers of "high fiber" granola bars sometimes create these bars by taking a fiber source, processing it heavily, and then adding it back in. We just don't know if your gut microbes like that fiber as much as the fiber in vegetables. Until we know more, you shouldn't rely solely on processed fiber.

4. "Gluten-free" processed foods. There appear to be rising rates of irritable bowel syndrome, gut dysbiosis, celiac disease, and gluten intolerance. That means many people are either required to (or are choosing to) avoid gluten. In response, we've seen a huge increase in the number of gluten-free (GF) foods available. Please be careful with these, because there's nothing magical about a gluten-free food. There are healthy GF foods, and there are unhealthy GF foods. Some are processed foods that are just as high in salt, sugar, and fat as their counterparts. It's up to you to read the nutritional labels and decide whether it's a healthy choice.

Also remember that there's nothing inherently "bad" about gluten. If you have no medical reason to avoid gluten, then you don't need to worry. Intact grains such as barley contain gluten AND a number of powerful nutrients.

5. There's good "all-natural" and there's bad "all-natural." I love natural treatments and approaches, but the words "all-natural" don't prove anything about safety, effectiveness, or risk of allergy. In fact, there are very few terms used on a label that guarantee a healthy product, whether that's skin care products or processed foods. The words "hypoallergenic", "for sensitive skin", and many others have no legal definition, which means they're often just marketing. And even if a product truly is "all-natural", it can still be bad for your skin. "Natural" encompasses everything from poison ivy to coconut oil to thousands of plants in between. When it comes to natural oils, some are wonderful while others may prove harmful. Bottom line: when it comes to all-natural, you still need to educate yourself.

6. Extreme diets. Please be careful about extreme dietary recommendations that are backed only by pseudoscience. Also be careful about diets that should be done only under medical supervision. There are potential side effects to many diets, from high protein diets (risk of kidney disease) to high fat diets (risk of diarrhea). There are also potential side effects with elimination diets (such as GF and dairy-free diets) because you're eliminating foods (loss of nutrients) and replacing those with something else (which may be nutrient-poor). And if you're not careful, juicing can become a fiber-elimination diet. Your dietary choices should always be customized for your medical profile.

CHAPTER 26
LIFESTYLE AND DERMATOLOGY

The Effects Of Stress On The Skin

All of us experience stress in our lives. It's unavoidable. And that stress causes actual physical changes within our body and skin.

The stress response system was designed to protect us from threats, and it works great in the short term. It helps you run away from predators: your heart pumps faster, your breathing speeds up, and your vision narrows. It's a beautifully coordinated system.

- When your brain perceives a stressful event, it activates the body's response system.
- One arm of that system is called the HPA axis: the hypothalamic – pituitary – adrenal axis. The brain (hypothalamus) send a message to a gland (the pituitary) which creates a hormone messenger that travels to a different gland (your adrenals) to activate the production of stress hormones (especially cortisol).
- Another arm of the system activates the sympathetic nervous system, leading to higher levels of adrenaline.

These stress hormones are very useful in times of danger, but they can be harmful over the long term. And in today's modern world, with your stress response often activated over long periods of time, your body can suffer.

Elevated Cortisol Can Lead To Fragile Skin, Fat Deposits, And Other Skin Changes

Dermatologists are very familiar with cortisol, one of the major stress hormones, because elevated cortisol impacts our skin and body in many ways. Some of these effects we know about from medical conditions. In a condition known as Cushing's syndrome, cortisol is produced in very large amounts. This large excess of cortisol can cause multiple skin-related effects.

- Fragile, thinning skin
- Stretch marks
- Acne
- Darkening of skin
- Excessive hair growth/loss
- "Moon" facies
- Back fat/ pot belly
- Muscle loss

Even in lesser amounts, excess stress hormones can impact our skin. In one study of young adults, stress made acne worse. In another study of students studying for final exams, stress led to impaired skin barrier repair. In yet another study, interview stress led to higher plasma cortisol levels and also caused impaired skin barrier repair.

One summary research paper looked at studies on the relationship between stress and the skin's ability to repair itself. In 17 research studies, stress was associated with either impaired wound healing or abnormal biomarkers that measured wound healing.

These are only the skin effects. Stress hormones create a snowball effect: they increase inflammation in the body and trigger other changes that ultimately impact many organ systems.

Controlling Cortisol And Other Stress Hormones Is Important, Which Means That Coping Strategies Are Critical

Stress is unavoidable, which means that you must have coping strategies in place. Multiple research studies have shown that the right coping strategies can actually decrease cortisol levels in the body. Some of these strategies also have direct benefits for your skin. From exercise, to mindfulness, to social connections, there are multiple actions that you can take to stabilize your body's response to stressful situations.

Your body will respond to stress. It's your job to stabilize and calm that response.

There are a number of ways to reduce stress and cope with stress, but it does require some dedication to start and follow through on these strategies.

These STRESS strategies can help.

Socialize/ **T**rees/**R**each/**E**xercise/**S**tillness/**S**leep

SOCIALIZE

Your friends keep you sane. They also keep you healthy.

When we talk about coping strategies for stress, social support is a major one. In fact, there's a much stronger recognition now among doctors about the importance of social relationships. That's why time spent socializing should be a priority, especially during times of stress (especially when life gets so hectic that it seems as though you don't have the time).

> In one summary study looking at the findings of 148 studies, it was estimated that people with stronger social relationships had a 50% increased likelihood of survival.

While there are many reasons behind this, social support has been linked to improved physical health. It's been linked to lower blood pressure, less inflammation, and even improved wound healing.

TREES

You may have sensed yourself feeling more calm and relaxed when surrounded by the forest. I grew up with a forest in my backyard (in the beautiful hills of Pittsburgh), and to this day hiking and spending time in nature are some of my favorite activities. Now researchers have documented, in study after study, that "forest therapy" actually results in measurable changes in the body's stress response.

In one study, both blood pressure and blood levels of the stress hormone cortisol were lower in middle-aged males when measured 2 hours after "forest therapy".

This activity simply involved several hours of walking around the forest and then sitting and lying down amongst the trees. This brief, simple activity resulted in measurable health benefits.

REACH

How do you live your life? Are you just trying to get to the weekend, or is there a deeper meaning and purpose in your life?

It's now recognized that reaching for a higher purpose in life may help keep you healthier. Volunteering to help others, for example, has been linked to better health. It's not known whether this is due to the reduction of stress hormones or whether it's because it impacts your other behaviors. But living your life with purpose has been linked to a reduced risk of heart disease, as well as death from all causes, even in those under chronic stress.

Living a life with purpose has been defined in different ways in the research studies. It may mean that you feel you have a purpose in life, or that you feel useful to family/friends/others/society, or that you have a system of values and beliefs that guide your daily activities.

Even just reaching for goals, such as via hobbies, can keep you healthier; one study found that patients who reported higher participation in enjoyable leisure activities had lower blood pressure and total cortisol levels.

EXERCISE

There's a reason why taking out your stress on a punching bag feels so great: it's a great way to burn off cortisol. Exercise is a great, highly effective tool to reduce levels of stress hormones.

Exercise has plenty of other skin benefits as well. It's definitely one of the keys to maintaining stable blood sugar levels. It may also help strengthen the skin, possibly by triggering the release of helpful substances from the muscles into the circulation.

In one experiment, previously inactive elderly adults began a 3-month cycling exercise program. Afterwards, their skin showed higher levels of collagen. Researchers believe that this may be due to certain hormones that are secreted by muscles during exercise. One of these substances, IL-15, has been shown in mice studies to impact the health of skin tissue.

STILLNESS

It's not always the days when you're running around that cause the most stress. It's often the days when you're sitting at a desk, and your mind is running around.

Frenzied thoughts (I need to respond to those 12 emails/2 voicemails/plan dinner/get a better phone plan/etc/etc) are enough to activate your body's stress response system.

That's why finding ways to slow down those frenzied thoughts (or finding ways to notice them but not react to them) can be so helpful to the body.

There's been lots of research over the last decade on the benefits of stillness in the form of meditation. Meditation often brings to mind an image of a person sitting cross-legged on the floor and maintaining a calm mind. While that's a very effective coping strategy, there are actually lots of ways to achieve a calmer mind and reduce your physical responses to stressful thoughts.

Prayer and gratitude prayers have been known for centuries. There's also a renewed appreciation for focusing on the body's movement to still the mind. Some experts call this moving meditation, and you may have felt it when you're running, swimming, or hiking.

One of my favorites is progressive muscle relaxation. That's a very fancy term for a very simple exercise that only takes a few minutes. There are plenty of apps that can guide you through a few minutes of first tensing, then relaxing, the different muscles in your body. (Focus on the body's movement to still the mind.)

Another easy, yet very effective technique, is simple breathing.

> Just practicing slow breathing exercises for three months resulted in lower blood pressure in a group of patients with hypertension. These patients also showed improvement in the autonomic nervous system.

The autonomic nervous system works outside of your conscious control. It can trigger the "fight or flight" response to stress, with an increased heart rate and faster breathing. In today's modern world, this system can be activated and stay that way, even in the absence of any direct threats.

Certain breathing exercises, practiced regularly, can help you balance out this response. One study found that regular breathing exercises, including slow breathing (for 3 months) and alternate nostril breathing (for 6 weeks), actually had measurable effects on the autonomic nervous system.

SLEEP

When our schedule gets overloaded, sleep is usually the first thing we cut. But as more and more research studies have found, that's not good.

Poor sleep been associated with significant health problems, including heart disease and diabetes. Studies have shown that getting less sleep (or just experiencing disturbed sleep) has been associated with higher levels of evening cortisol.

Poor sleep also has direct, measurable effects on the skin, including the skin's repair systems.

Your skin has a remarkable ability to repair itself. But poor sleep weakens that ability. In one study, researchers damaged the skin barrier of volunteers. Those who reported poor sleep repaired the skin damage more slowly than the good sleepers. When the poor sleepers were exposed to UV radiation, their skin also took longer to recover from the resulting sunburn.

The findings went even deeper than that. In patients reporting poor quality sleep, their skin showed more signs of aging, including uneven pigmentation and reduced elasticity.

Section 4

RECIPES

Tying It All Together: Skin Saving Foods + Recipes

You have the potential to power up just about every meal of your day. From breakfast to soups to snacks, there are ways to add powerful skin saving ingredients to just about every meal.

The recipes in this section are meant to help you do just that. They meet the 3 major goals of eating for younger skin: They add in many powerful nutrients. They're designed to limit sugar spikes. And they avoid deep-fried and heavily processed foods.

Healthy Cooking: Ideas and Suggestions

Under skin saving sides, you'll find a recipe for roasted Brussels sprouts. I love all the crispy Brussels sprouts I'm seeing on appetizer menus. These are simple to re-create at home. You can chop the sprouts in under 5 minutes (just chop in half), and the rest of the recipe is just a shake and bake: shake on the flavors, gently combine, and bake in the oven.

This recipe really highlights one important point: the hardest part of cooking vegetables isn't the difficulty factor. It's the learning how and the planning how.

- You have to learn how to best maximize taste and looks and nutrition.
- And you have to learn how to plan a weekly menu, because only the super-experienced can come home, look in the fridge, and on-the-spot cook up a tasty, nutritious dinner.

In the sections that follow, you'll find mostly straightforward recipes, with a few more complex recipes sprinkled in.

Personally, I used to be intimidated by certain recipes with their long lists of ingredients. Once I started to deconstruct recipes (break down them into their basic techniques), many of them seemed much more doable. For the recipes that follow, even if you have minimal cooking experience, you'll still be able to handle most of the techniques involved.

- **Power blends.** Just blend the ingredients
- **Shake and bake.** Shake on some flavorings and bake
- **Toss it and top it.** Just like a salad: toss your ingredients together and then add a topping
- **Boil.** Several recipes involve boiling, but if you can boil pasta, then you can cook lentils and quinoa.
- **Sauté and simmer.** If you can boil pasta, then you can sauté and simmer. To sauté, just heat some oil, add your ingredients, and cook for a few minutes by stirring. To simmer, boil gently.

Heritage Diets

A number of these recipes are derived from traditional heritage foods: tomato herb salad, gazpacho, Romesco sauce, turmeric yogurt with roasted Indian spices, and others. Heritage diets are a wonderful place to look for recipes for a whole foods diet. Many of the world's traditional cuisines were (by necessity) based on whole foods. And over many years, these chefs have learned how to maximize flavor, appearance, and often health benefits.

Whole Foods and Healthy Shortcuts

These recipes are centered around whole foods (ingredients that are close to their natural form) and lightly processed foods. That doesn't mean you'll be lunching on raw carrots; it just means a focus on foods that aren't heavily processed. This includes a range of foods, because certain processing techniques make foods safer to eat or increase shelf life without depleting nutrients. A whole foods diet can incorporate plenty of cooked, frozen, and canned foods.

When you're trying to decide if a particular product fits into a whole foods diet, you really have to rely on the ingredient list (what have they added to those carrots?) as well as the nutrition facts label (how much added sugar is in that green tea?). Don't rely on the label found on the front of the package, because many of those focus on marketing claims.

As for healthy cooking, I'm always on the lookout for nutritious, time-saving shortcuts, whether that's the right gadgets or the right pre-prepped foods. I use certain foods all the time, because they make healthy cooking so much easier: frozen fruits and vegetables (without added sugar, salt, or fat), canned beans (rinsed before using), pouches of salmon and cans of tuna, and nut butters. Another time-saving tactic is cooking, then freezing, whole grains and dried beans.

As with everything else, getting better at cooking tasty + healthy food requires some know-how and a lot of practice. Some cooking schools, stores and restaurants offer classes focused on healthy cooking or healthy traditional cuisines. These classes may even be offered at your medical center.

The Tulane University Goldring Center for Culinary Medicine has been expanding their program to other centers under the direction of Dr. Timothy Harlan. In Houston, we now have the Nourish Program at the University of Texas School of Public Health. These programs offer classes to the public. They also train professionals in culinary medicine, which combines nutrition and culinary knowledge to achieve optimal health.

Naperville Public Library

Try our mobile app available for iOS and Android devices. 630-961-4100

Check out receipt

Date: 3/16/2024 4:47:04 PM

1. **Four ways to beat the market : a practical guide to stock-screening strategies to help you pick winn**
Barcode 31318059325547
Due by 4/6/2024

2. **Glow : the dermatologist's guide to a whole foods younger skin diet / Rajani Katta, M.D.**
Barcode 31318049257503
Due by 4/6/2024

3. **The little book of money : a guide to managing your finances, building your wealth, and investing in**
Barcode 31318059265511
Due by 4/6/2024

CHAPTER 27
SKIN SAVING STARTS

BREAKFAST TACOS

SPINACH FRITTATA

OVERNIGHT COCOA BANANA OATS

PALEO BREAKFAST TART

If you picture the standard American breakfast, you're not seeing much in the way of fruits and vegetables. (And if you're a child of the 80s, your breakfast was probably Froot Loops, not fruit.)

You can power up breakfast pretty easily, though. These recipes add hefty doses of protein, fiber, and produce.

High Protein, High Produce Breakfasts: Spinach Frittata and Breakfast Taco For those who are carb-sensitive, starting the day with a high protein breakfast may be helpful. Breakfast tacos are a high protein start, and they can be easily customized. You can scramble your eggs with just about any vegetable: in my family, we've done fresh spinach or butternut squash puree, although my favorite is sautéed onions, peppers, and cilantro. Frittatas are another great base for adding in vegetables. They're an easy way to add in spinach, but you can easily substitute any chopped vegetable.

A Touch of Sweet: Breakfast Tarts and Oatmeal For family members who prefer a touch of sweet, the bananas and blueberries in the breakfast tart add a little sweet, along with fiber and antioxidant polyphenols. (Although it's a bit sweet, it's still a lower carb option for those who are sensitive). For a higher-carb breakfast, oatmeal adds in a nice dose of prebiotic fiber, while adding in almond butter (healthy fats) and chia seeds (fiber) helps to stabilize the blood sugar response. Adding in cocoa powder, nuts, and bananas means extra antioxidants and fiber.

Spinach Frittata

The Basics: Sauté then bake
Yield: 4 servings | Prep time: 5 min | Cooking time: 15 min

Ingredients

2 tbsp olive oil
1 onion, diced
2 cloves garlic, minced
10 oz frozen chopped spinach, thawed (or fresh)
6 eggs

Herbs/spices

1 tsp basil
1 tsp oregano
3/4 tsp salt

Topping

1/4 cup feta cheese

Directions

1. Preheat oven to 400°
2. Heat oil in oven-safe skillet
3. Sauté onion until softened, about 3 minutes
4. Add garlic cloves and spinach and sauté for another 3 minutes
5. In bowl, whisk together eggs and seasonings
6. Pour egg mixture over vegetables and cook until almost set, about 5 minutes
7. Top with feta cheese and transfer to oven
8. Cook for 5 to 8 minutes, until puffed

Breakfast Tacos

The Basics: Sauté then scramble
Yield: 4 servings | Prep time: 10 min | Cooking time: 10 min

Ingredients

Main Ingredients
2 tbsp olive oil
1 onion, diced
1 large tomato, diced
1/2 red bell pepper, diced
1 clove garlic, minced
1 tsp smoked paprika
1 tsp turmeric
1/2 tsp salt (or to taste)
1/4 tsp pepper (or to taste)
1/4 bunch cilantro (leaves and stems, tough ends discarded)
4 eggs, whisked

For serving
4 tortillas, corn or flour
Shredded cheese (optional)

Directions

1. Heat oil on medium heat in large skillet
2. Add onions, vegetables, garlic, and spices
3. Sauté until onions soften, about 3-5 minutes
4. Add cilantro
5. Add eggs and cook, stirring to scramble, until done, about 3 minutes
6. Add eggs to tortilla, top with cheese if desired, and fold over

Overnight Cocoa Banana Oats

The Basics: Mix and refrigerate
Yield: 1 serving | Prep time: 5 min | Cooking time: Overnight

Ingredients

1/2 cup milk (dairy or non-dairy)
1/2 tbsp chai seeds
1 tbsp cocoa powder
1 tsp honey (or to taste)
1/2 cup old-fashioned rolled oats
1 tbsp almond butter
Half a banana, sliced
1/2 tbsp chopped walnuts

Directions

1. Mix together first 4 ingredients in jar (with lid), or in bowl
2. Add oats and stir to combine
3. Add almond butter and stir in gently
4. Cover tightly and let sit in fridge overnight
5. Top with banana and walnuts

Breakfast Tarts

The Basics: Mix batter and bake
Yield: 2 servings | Prep time: 5 min | Cooking time: 10 min

Ingredients

3 eggs
2 ripe bananas, mashed
6 tbsp shredded coconut, unsweetened
1 tsp cinnamon

Topping

1/2 cup blueberries, fresh or frozen (partially thawed)

Directions

1. Preheat oven to 400°
2. Mix all ingredients
3. Prepare tart pans: spray cooking spray on 3" tart pans (6 pans)
4. Spoon 2 tbsp batter into each pan
5. Bake for 10 minutes
6. Serve topped with blueberries

Cooking Notes: If you don't have tart pans, these can be cooked on the stovetop. Cook as you would pancakes: spoon batter onto hot skillet (greased with cooking spray) and cook for about 3 minutes each side.

CHAPTER 28
SKIN SAVING SNACKS

CRISPY CHICKPEAS

HUMMUS WITH PEPPER STRIPS AND PITA CHIPS

LAYERED VEGGIE DIP

RED BEAN MUSHROOM FRITTERS

ANTS ON A LOG

It's a long way from lunch to dinner, and you may feel your blood sugar dropping around that 3-4 pm mark. (That's when I personally feel the call of the vending machine.) Those vending machine snacks just don't have staying power, though. I'm ravenous by the time dinner comes around, thanks to the sugar spike roller coaster.

Snacks like the following ones, which help stabilize blood sugar with either protein or fiber, can help.

Crispy Chickpeas Crispy chickpeas are simple: shake and bake. They taste especially good straight from the oven, with a wonderful texture--crispy outside, creamy inside.

Chickpeas: Protein and Fiber Rich I'm always looking for more ways to add beans and lentils to our diet, because they're a great source of energy-rich carbs, combined with a hefty dose of both protein and fiber. A 1 cup serving of chickpeas provides close to 15 grams of protein. (In comparison, one egg provides 6 grams of protein.) It also provides over 12 grams of fiber, which gets you close to half of the recommended amount of 25 grams of fiber a day for women.

Hummus: Nutrient-Dense Hummus is what I call a power blend: start with a few powerhouse ingredients and then blend. It's become a popular dip, and for good reason: it's tasty, it's easy to make (or buy), and it's packed with nutrients. In fact, one study compared the nutrient density of different dips (via the Naturally Nutrient Rich score, which looks at nutrient-to-calorie ratios). Hummus was the top-scoring dip, scoring significantly higher than ranch dressing and cream cheese.

Minerals in Hummus While chickpeas are a great source of protein and fiber, they also provide a nice dose of iron and zinc, both important nutrients for hair growth. Chickpeas also provide a hefty dose of folate, important in cell repair, as well as other minerals such as manganese and copper.

Power Fats in Hummus Tahini adds the creaminess to hummus, and it's made from ground sesame seeds: I think of tahini as sesame seed butter (just like peanut butter is made from ground peanuts). In addition to PUFAs, it provides an extra dose of B vitamins and minerals, along with phytonutrients such as sesame seed lignans. Even the olive oil (MUFAs), lemon juice (extra boost of vitamin C), and garlic provide extra benefits.

Carrot Sticks and Pepper Strips: Extra Nutrients If you serve hummus with carrot sticks and red pepper strips, even better: carrots provide beta-carotene and fiber, while red pepper are a great source of vitamin C. That vitamin C has an extra benefit: it helps your body absorb the iron in the chickpeas.

Layered Veggie Dip: Antioxidants This layered dip serves up even more antioxidants, from the sweet potatoes (beta-carotene) and black beans (anthocyanins) to the tomatoes (lycopene).

Red Bean Mushroom Fritters: A High Protein Snack Red bean mushroom fritters is another snack that's surprisingly nutritious for being so tasty. Just like crabcakes, you can serve them as an appetizer or on a bed of salad greens, although they do taste best when served fresh from the skillet. These fritters pack in 3 vegetables, which means they pack a lot of nutrients in a small package. Just 1 cup of cooked kidney beans provides about 15 grams of protein.

Kidney Beans and Carrots: Antioxidant-Rich Kidney beans also supply antioxidants, including the anthocyanins which give these beans their red color. In fact, studies of the antioxidant capacity of different fruits and vegetables have found that beans are among the best sources. Carrots provide more power: they're a great source of carotenoids, the red-orange pigments that function as strong antioxidants and are converted by the body to vitamin A, important for cell turnover and skin renewal.

Mushrooms: Low Calorie, High Flavor As for mushrooms, I'm always trying to add them to recipes, because they're low calorie but high flavor, especially when cooked in a little olive oil. They're a good source of prebiotic fiber as well as vitamins and minerals, including several B vitamins and selenium, another strong antioxidant.

Ants on a Log: Low Calorie, Fights Collagen Damage As for ants on a log, I had to include it because although it's been around forever, it's experiencing a resurgence. Celery sticks are a great low-calorie snack, and they actually provide a nice boost of fiber and other phytonutrients. They're a source of luteolin and apigenin, compounds which fight off the collagen-degrading enzyme collagenase. Peanut butter is a great source of MUFAs, providing some staying power to this snack and an extra benefit to your skin barrier.

Crispy Spicy Chickpeas

The Basics: Shake and bake
Yield: 4 servings | Prep time: 5 min | Cooking time: 25 min

Ingredients

1 can chickpeas (also known as garbanzo beans), rinsed and drained (15 oz can)
1 tbsp olive oil
1 tsp brown sugar
1/2 tsp salt
1/2 tsp smoked paprika
1/4 tsp ground cumin

Directions

1. Preheat oven to 400°
2. Mix all ingredients together
3. Place on a roasting pan in a single layer. For easier clean-up, line the pan with foil or parchment paper
4. Bake for 25 minutes

Hummus with Carrot Sticks and Pepper Strips

The Basics: Blend
Yield: 4 servings | Prep time: 5 min | Cooking time: 1 min

Ingredients

1 can chickpeas, rinsed and drained [15 oz]
1/4 cup lemon juice
2 tbsp tahini
2 tbsp extra-virgin olive oil
2 tbsp water
1 clove garlic, peeled
1/2 tsp salt [or to taste]

To serve: 2 tsp olive oil, 1 tsp smoked paprika, few whole chickpeas

Directions

1. Add garlic to food processor and mince
2. Add all other ingredients and blend well
3. Garnish with olive oil, paprika, and whole chickpeas
4. Serve alongside carrot sticks and pepper strips (red, orange, or yellow bell peppers cored and sliced into strips)

Layered Veggie Dip

The Basics: Microwave potato, then assemble
Yield: 4 servings | Prep time: 5 min | Cooking time: 8 min

Ingredients

1 sweet potato, medium
1 can black beans (15 oz), drained and rinsed
1/2 tsp basil
1/2 tsp oregano
1 cup cherry tomatoes, sliced in half
1/2 cup loosely packed Romaine lettuce, shredded
2 tbsp shredded cheese (optional)

Directions

1. Cook sweet potato: wash, poke several times with fork, then microwave for 6 minutes. Once cooled, remove flesh from skin and coarsely mash. Spoon into 4 tall glasses
2. Mash black beans in a bowl with basil and oregano and then add to glasses
3. Add layer of chopped cherry tomatoes
4. Add layer of shredded romaine lettuce
5. Top with shredded cheese (optional)
6. Serve with carrot sticks, red pepper strips, or toasted tortilla strips

Red Bean Mushroom Fritters

The Basics: Cook in skillet
Yield: 4 servings | Prep time: 10 min | Cooking time: 10 min

Ingredients

1 can (15 oz) dark red kidney beans, rinsed and drained
6 oz cremini or portabello mushrooms, chopped
1 cup carrots, shredded
1 cup rolled oats [old-fashioned]
1 egg, beaten
1 tsp salt
1 tsp paprika
1 tsp soy sauce [low sodium]
2 tbsp tomato paste

2 tbsp olive oil

Directions

1. Coarsely mash kidney beans
2. Add in all other ingredients (except for olive oil) and mix well
3. Form into small patties
4. Let sit in fridge for 30 minutes (to help fritters maintain shape when cooking)
5. Heat 2 tbsp olive oil in skillet on medium heat
6. Cook fritters 3-5 minutes (until brown), then flip and cook on other side
7. Transfer to plate, and repeat with remaining fritters

Ants On A Log

The Basics: Assemble
Yield: 2 servings | Prep time: 5 min | Cooking time: 1 min

Ingredients

4 celery stalks (may peel if preferred), each chopped into
about 3 pieces
4 tbsp peanut butter
2 tbsp raisins

Directions

1. Spread peanut butter on celery sticks
2. Sprinkle with raisins

CHAPTER 29
SKIN SAVING SIPPERS

GREEN TEA

CHAI TEA

GINGER TEA

GREEN SMOOTHIE

Plain, filtered tap water is a great beverage. I avoid plastic water bottles, but I carry my glass or stainless steel water bottles, filled with water from the fridge, everywhere. It's important to stay well-hydrated, since dehydration leads to fatigue and other problems. It also accentuates fine lines and wrinkles. While the proper level of hydration is important, be aware that overhydration won't solve dry skin or skin inflammation.

How much water should you drink? This may vary from day to day, depending on how much fluid you're taking in from fruits, vegetables, and other beverages, and how much you're losing, such as in sweat. As a general rule of thumb, if you're experiencing thirst, dry mouth, or dark yellow urine, you need to increase your fluid intake.

For extra nutrients, flavor, and variety throughout your day, these beverages are other options.

Green and Black Tea: Potent Antioxidants The catechins in tea leaves are potent antioxidants. Both black tea and green tea are great sources of these powerful phytonutrients. (Some studies have shown equivalent effects of black tea and green tea. In one study, for example, they were almost equally beneficial in preventing skin cancers in mice exposed to UV radiation. Other research has found higher antioxidant levels in green tea.) Other types of tea also have powerful benefits, including white tea, sencha tea, and matcha tea. If you're sensitive to caffeine, feel free to go caffeine-free. Research has found that decaffeinated versions have beneficial effects as well, although they may be slightly less effective.

Chai Tea: Spices Add More Power Chai tea is very popular in India. While there are many different versions, a key feature is the use of antioxidant and anti-inflammatory spices.

Ginger Tea: Anti-Inflammatory Ginger is known for its anti-inflammatory abilities, and ginger extract has even shown promise in fighting off the scissor enzyme elastase. This tea is a simple way to get a small dose of ginger's benefits.

Green Smoothie: A Dose of Spinach and Pineapple While you have to be very careful when it comes to smoothies (many are loaded with added sugar) this option provides an easy dose of spinach and pineapple. Do be warned, though: even with the pineapple, it's not that sweet, especially if you're used to smoothies from a kiosk or fast-food restaurant. (It can take a while to retrain your taste buds, but once they've been retrained, many people find fast-food drinks too sweet).

Other Beverages: Infused Waters and Probiotic Drinks Infused water is another easy way to add in a few extra nutrients and flavor. For one option, fill your bottle with mint leaves and cucumber slices, and then add water. I've seen lots of creative combinations, and I like water with mint leaves and frozen berries. Another beverage option: probiotic beverages such as kombucha (fermented tea) and kefir (a fermented dairy beverage). Just be careful with the purchased types. I've looked at many labels, and some of these have very high levels of added sugar.

Green Tea

The Basics: Boil water
Yield: 1 serving | Prep time: 1 min | Cooking time: 8 min

Ingredients

1 green tea bag or 1 tsp loose-leaf green tea
1 cup fresh water
Sweetener, to taste

Directions

1. Place tea bag in cup; if using loose-leaf, put tea in an infuser basket and then place in cup
2. Boil water
3. Let water rest for 1-2 minutes to cool down slightly
4. Pour water over tea
5. Let steep 2-3 minutes
6. Remove tea bag (or leaves) and serve

Chai Tea

The Basics: Boil (water+milk+spices), then add tea bags
Yield: 4 servings | Prep time: 5 min | Cooking time: 12 min

Ingredients

2 cups milk (dairy or non-dairy)
2 cups water
Ginger, 1" piece (peeled and grated on large holes of grater)
3 cinnamon sticks
8 cloves
8 cardamom pods
4 black tea bags

Directions

1. Crush cardamom pods with back of spoon
2. Pour water, milk, and all spices into sauce pan
3. Bring to a boil, then remove from heat
4. Add tea bags and steep for 10 minutes
5. Remove tea bags, strain out spices, and pour into 4 cups
6. Sweeten to taste

Cooking Notes: There are many variations of chai, and this recipe can be easily customized. You can adjust the quantity of milk, as well as the type and quantity of spices.

Ginger Tea

The Basics: Boil water and grate ginger
Yield: 2 servings | Prep time: 3 min | Cooking time: 12 min

Ingredients

1 knob of ginger root
2 cups water
2 tsp sweetener (or to taste)

Directions

1. Peel ginger root (peels easily using the edge of a spoon)
2. Grate peeled ginger, using the large holes of a grater
3. Place 1/2 tsp of grated ginger in each cup (use more for spicier tea)
4. Boil water, then pour over ginger
5. Steep for 10 minutes
6. Strain out ginger, add sweetener to taste, and serve

Green Smoothie

The Basics: Blend
Yield: 2 servings | Prep time: 2 min | Cooking time: 2 min

Ingredients

2 cups (loosely packed) fresh baby spinach leaves
1 cup frozen pineapple chunks, partially thawed
1 cup water

Directions

1. Place ingredients in blender or food processor
2. Blend until smooth
3. If needed, may add 1 tsp honey (or to taste)

CHAPTER 30
SKIN SAVING SALADS

SPINACH/STRAWBERRY/BALSAMIC VINAIGRETTE/WALNUTS

TOMATO HERB SALAD

SPICE RICE POWER BOWL

QUINOA SALAD

Salads: The Perfect Base to Add in Power-Packed Ingredients I love salads, because you can start with a base that's a nutritional powerhouse, and then add in multiple other powerful ingredients. From the base, to the main ingredients, to the crunchy toppings, to the dressing, each and every salad component can be designed for maximum nutrient power.

Spinach Salad: A Powerhouse Base A basic spinach salad is a great example of this principle. You start with a nutritional powerhouse base: baby spinach leaves. Then you add in extras that boost the nutrient profile, including strawberries and toasted walnuts. With a balsamic vinaigrette, you can choose a power fat (extra virgin olive oil) and a high-quality balsamic vinegar (to add in polyphenols).

Tomato Herb Salad: Two Potent Skin-Saving Foods Combined This is a basic recipe, but it provides some potent benefits. With lycopene and other nutrients, tomatoes have potent skin saving abilities. With the olive oil, vinegar, and herbs adding in additional benefits, this simple salad is surprisingly helpful.

Spice Rice Power Bowl: Power Carbs, Vegetables, And Spices
Grain salads make for easy sides. They can also be easily customized to create entrée salads by adding a healthy protein source, such as tofu, chickpeas, or a healthy seafood or meat. Brown rice as the base means a whole grain with plenty of fiber and antioxidants. Plenty of herbs and spices (along with onions, ginger, and garlic) means a powerful dose of antioxidants, while the vegetables add another strong dose of phytonutrients with antioxidant and prebiotic benefits.

Quinoa Salad: Packed with Phytonutrients Quinoa is a power carb, with a hefty serving of protein, fiber, vitamins, and minerals. The extras in this salad are packed with phytonutrients, from the carrots to the red peppers to the chopped apples.

Extra Nutrients: Pumpkin Seeds, Olive Oil, and Vinegar Adding in herbs and spices packs in more antioxidant and anti-inflammatory phytonutrients, while the pumpkin seeds add in healthy fat and extra zinc. Even the salad dressing adds in extra nutrients: olive oil (in moderation) may aid skin elasticity, while the live cultures in apple cider vinegar (look for them on the label) are a probiotic.

Spinach Strawberry Salad with Balsamic Dressing

The Basics: Toss it and top it
Yield: 2 servings | Prep time: 10 min | Cooking time: 5 min

Ingredients

4 cups fresh baby spinach leaves
1 cup fresh strawberries, hulled and quartered
1/2 red bell pepper, diced
1/4 cup walnut halves

Dressing

2 tbsp extra virgin olive oil
1 tbsp aged balsamic vinegar
1 tsp Dijon mustard
1/4 tsp salt (or to taste)

Directions

1. Toast walnuts: place in dry skillet over medium heat, and stir until fragrant (about 3-4 minutes)
2. Make dressing: Place ingredients in a jar with tight lid, and shake to combine
3. Place salad ingredients in serving bowl and serve with dressing on the side

Tomato Herb Salad

The Basics: Toss it and top it
Yield: 6 servings | Prep time: 5 min | Cooking time: 1 min

Ingredients

1 lb multicolored cherry tomatoes, sliced in half
2 tbsp extra virgin olive oil
1 tbsp apple cider vinegar (or any flavored vinegar with live
    cultures)
1 tsp sugar
1 tsp dried oregano
1/2 tsp salt

Topping

2 tbsp fresh basil leaves, chopped
2 tbsp fresh mint leaves, chopped

Directions

1. Place tomatoes in a bowl
2. Make dressing: Place all other ingredients in a jar with
   tight lid, and shake to combine
3. Add dressing to tomatoes, and gently stir
4. Chill in refrigerator until ready to serve
5. When ready to serve, garnish with fresh herbs

Spice Rice Power Bowl

The Basics: Sauté flavor base, then vegetables, then combine
Yield: 6 servings | Prep time: 10 min | Cooking time: 15 min

Ingredients

Flavor Base
2 tablespoons ghee or olive oil
1 onion, chopped
3 garlic cloves, minced
Ginger, 2" piece (peeled and grated on large holes of grater)
1/2 cup unsalted roasted cashews
2 cinnamon sticks, broken into large pieces
1 tbsp cardamom pods

Main ingredients
1 lb frozen mixed vegetables, thawed
2 tsp garam masala (homemade or purchased)
1/4 bunch chopped cilantro (leaves and stems, tough ends discarded)
1 tsp salt (may add more to taste)
1 pinch saffron, soaked in 1 tsp water

2 cups cooked brown rice

Directions

1. Heat oil on medium in large skillet
2. Sauté flavor base: onion, ginger, garlic, cashews, cinnamon, and cardamom, until onions soften
3. Add all other ingredients (except for rice) and cook, stirring occasionally, until flavors have combined, about 5 to 8 minutes
4. Transfer to large serving bowl and add rice. Stir gently to combine.

Quinoa Salad

The Basics: Boil quinoa, then toss it and top it
Yield: 6 servings | Prep time: 10 min | Cooking time: 20 min

Ingredients

1 cup quinoa, uncooked, rinsed well
2 cups water
1/2 cup shredded carrots
1/2 cup cooked chickpeas (if canned, rinse well)
1/2 cup chopped apples
1/2 cup chopped red bell pepper

Dressing

3 tbsp apple cider vinegar
1 tbsp extra virgin olive oil
1/2 tsp salt
1/4 tsp black pepper

Topping

1/4 cup chopped cilantro (leaves and stems, tough ends
discarded)
1/4 cup toasted pumpkin seeds

Directions

1. Add quinoa and water to saucepan and bring to full boil
2. Lower heat to low, cover pan, and cook for 15 minutes
3. Remove pot from heat and let stand for 5 minutes
4. While quinoa is cooking, make dressing: place dressing ingredients in a jar with tight lid, and shake to combine
5. Transfer cooked quinoa to serving bowl and fluff with fork. Add other ingredients and dressing and stir gently
6. Top with cilantro and pumpkin seeds

CHAPTER 31
SKIN SAVING SOUPS

LENTIL STEW

FOUR-VEGGIE TEXAS CHILI

GOLDEN YOGURT WITH ROASTED SPICES

GAZPACHO

Starting a meal with soup is a simple way to add more vegetables to a meal. Soups are also great if you're making after school snacks for the children. If you invest in a thermos, they also make for a great take-to-work meal.

Gazpacho: Pack In Vegetables Most soups are easy opportunities to pack in more vegetables. Gazpacho is known for being a refreshing, chilled soup, and it's simple to make. Gazpacho is essentially just a simple power blend of fresh, ripe vegetables. With tomatoes, cucumbers, and peppers, garnished with herbs, this simple blend packs in multiple phytonutrients.

Lentil Stew: High-Fiber With savory lentil stew, you're packing in lentils, carrots, onions, and tomatoes. If you're not used to cooking with lentils, you might be surprised to find out how easy they are. They don't require any pre-soaking, so you can just pour them from a bag right into your soup. If you can boil pasta, then you can cook lentils. One cup of cooked lentils contains 16 g of dietary fiber, which makes it an outstanding source of fiber. (That's almost half of the 38 grams recommended for men daily.)

That healthy dose of fiber and protein in lentils has been shown to help regulate blood sugar levels. A study published in the *Archives of Internal Medicine* studied the effects of adding legumes to the diet of persons with diabetes. Eating just one extra cup of legumes daily led to improvements in blood sugar, as well as improvements in cholesterol and triglycerides.

Veggie Chili: Packed With Antioxidants With veggie chili, you're getting a strong dose of multiple antioxidants. Lycopene in particular (from tomatoes) has been shown to help protect against skin damage following UV radiation. Onions, spices, black beans, kidney beans, and bulgur are also all great sources of antioxidants.

Whole Grain Bulgur Bulgur is an easy addition: it cooks right in the chili, so there are no extra steps or dishes. Bulgur is a type of whole grain wheat, with many intact nutrients. It's essentially a type of pre-cooked wheat. Only the outermost layer of the wheat kernels are removed, which leaves most of the nutrients in the wheat intact. These kernels are then partially cooked, dried, and broken into pieces. This means that while bulgur is still a whole grain, it cooks fairly quickly.

Golden Yogurt: Probiotics, Prebiotics, And Antioxidants In One Recipe Yogurt with live, active cultures is a great probiotic. This recipe turns it into an antioxidant-packed probiotic. How? By adding potent antioxidant spices, including turmeric, coriander seeds, and cumin seeds. The addition of tomatoes and onions means extra antioxidants and a dose of prebiotics as well.

Savory Lentil Stew

The Basics: Sauté and simmer
Yield: 8 servings | Prep time: 5 min | Cooking time: 25 min

Ingredients

Flavor base
2 tbsp olive oil
1 onion, diced
2 carrots, chopped

Main ingredients
1 cup French green lentils
4 cup water
2 tsp soy sauce [low-sodium]
2 tbsp tomato paste

Herbs/Spices
1 tsp salt
1/2 tsp each: thyme, black pepper, garlic powder
1/4 tsp cumin

Directions

1. Heat oil on medium-high heat
2. Sauté onions and carrots until onions are translucent
3. Add lentils and water
4. Add spices, soy sauce, and tomato paste
5. Bring to a boil, then reduce heat and simmer, covered, for 20 minutes

Four Veggie Texas Chili

The Basics: Sauté and simmer
Yield: 8 servings | Prep time: 5 min | Cooking time: 15 min

Ingredients

Flavor Base
2 tbsp olive oil
1 onion, chopped
1/2 cup golden raisins

Sauce
1 8oz can tomato sauce
2 tsp apple cider vinegar

Spices
2 tsp each: basil/ oregano/ garlic powder
1 tsp each: salt/ cumin
1/2 tsp chili powder
1 bay leaf

Main chili ingredients
1 16oz can red kidney beans, rinsed and drained
1 15oz can black beans, rinsed and drained
1/2 cup bulgur
1 cup water

Directions
1. Heat oil in saucepan on medium-high heat, then add onions and sauté until golden
2. Add raisins, tomato sauce, vinegar, and spices. Cook 2 minutes, stirring occasionally
3. Add main ingredients and lower heat to low. Cook, covered, for 10 minutes, stirring occasionally

Golden Yogurt

The Basics: Sauté base, then add to yogurt
Yield: 4 servings | Prep time: 5 min | Cooking time: 12 min

Ingredients

1 tbsp olive oil
1/2 tbsp cumin seeds (whole)
1/2 tbsp coriander seeds (whole)
1 tomato, chopped
1 onion, chopped
1 tsp turmeric
1/4 tsp salt
1/4 tsp black pepper
8 oz of yogurt (with live active cultures)

Directions

1. In skillet, add olive oil, cumin seeds, and coriander seeds
2. Heat to medium, stirring frequently, for 1-2 minutes
3. When spices are fragrant, add tomatoes, onions, turmeric, salt, and pepper
4. Cook for 10 minutes, stirring occasionally
5. Add mixture to yogurt and gently combine

Gazpacho

The Basics: Blend
Yield: 4 servings | Prep time: 5 min | Cooking time: 2 min

Ingredients

3 large tomatoes (ripe), coarsely chopped
1/2 red bell pepper, coarsely chopped
1/2 small cucumber, peeled and seeded, coarsely chopped
1 garlic clove, pressed
2 tbsp extra virgin olive oil
1 tbsp sherry vinegar
1/2 tsp salt (or to taste)

Directions

1. Using food processor, puree tomatoes
2. Add all other ingredients and process until smooth
3. Thin with water if needed
4. Chill for at least 1 hour

CHAPTER 32
SKIN SAVING SAUCES

ROMESCO SAUCE

BASIL PESTO

MINT-CILANTRO CHUTNEY

HERB TAHINI SAUCE

I consider sauces a bonus food. With the right ones, you get a bonus boost of nutrients in your meal. In these recipes, the sauces provide a boost of vegetables and nuts (Romesco sauce), or herbs (mint-cilantro chutney), or herbs and nuts/seeds (basil pesto and herb tahini sauce).

Romesco Sauce: Beta-Carotene and Power Fats I've seen this sauce served on top of grilled chicken and fish. I've used it myself as an appetizer dip, served along with roasted cauliflower (a great skin-saving snack in its own right).

With roasted red peppers, tomato paste, and paprika, it provides a nice boost of powerful antioxidants. The almonds and olive oil provide a nice boost of power fats, which (in moderation) may help improve skin hydration and reduce skin sensitivity.

Basil Pesto: Strong Dose of Phytonutrients Herbs and spices in particular are concentrated sources of nutrients. In this recipe, the main ingredient is basil, a delicious herb that has the added bonus of containing high levels of certain flavonoids, strongly antioxidant compounds. The walnuts and extra-virgin olive oil provide a boost of omega-3 fatty acids and monounsaturated fatty acids.

Pesto can add a boost of flavor and nutrients to many different foods. I use it in place of mayonnaise on sandwiches, and it adds a nice depth of flavor when added to cooked vegetables. It can also be added to pasta, to cooked grains, or to a casserole. One of my favorite uses is as a topping for roasted salmon.

Mint-Cilantro Chutney: Packed with Herbs and Spices This bright green dipping sauce is a fixture in Indian restaurants, served alongside samosas. But it's not just for samosas; it can be used alongside many foods, as a dipping sauce or a topping or a dressing for a power grain bowl. This sauce, just like pesto, showcases herbs that are a concentrated source of nutrients.

Herb Tahini Sauce: Power Fats And More Herbs Another versatile sauce that provides a nice boost of herbs, along with tahini, the same creamy sesame seed butter that gives hummus its lovely texture.

Romesco Sauce

The Basics: Toast, then blend
Yield: 6 servings | Prep time: 1 min | Cooking time: 6 min

Ingredients

1 slice bread
1/4 cup sliced almonds
1 roasted red pepper (if using from jar, drain first)
2 tbsp tomato paste
1 tbsp sherry vinegar (or substitute other vinegar, such as
   apple cider)
1/2 tbsp paprika
1/4 tsp salt
2 tbsp extra virgin olive oil

Directions

1. Toast bread and almonds. You can toast in a toaster oven, or bake for 400° for 4-5 minutes (stirring almonds occasionally)
2. After toasting, add to food processor
3. Add all other ingredients and process

Basil Pesto

The Basics: Toast, then blend
Yield: 8 servings | Prep time: 5 min | Cooking time: 6 min

Ingredients

1 garlic clove, peeled
1/3 cup chopped walnuts
2 cups of basil leaves [loosely packed]
1/4 tsp salt
1/4 cup extra virgin olive oil
Optional: 1/4 cup grated Parmesan cheese

Directions

1. Toast walnuts and garlic: Heat skillet on medium-high, add walnuts and garlic clove, and heat for a few minutes, stirring frequently.
2. Add garlic, walnuts, basil and salt to food processor, and coarsely chop.
3. Add olive oil and process to the consistency of a thick paste.
4. If desired, add cheese and mix to combine

Mint-Cilantro Chutney

The Basics: Blend
Yield: 8 servings | Prep time: 5 min | Cooking time: 5 min

Ingredients

1 cup, packed, fresh cilantro, coarsely chopped
   (both leaves and stems, with tough ends discarded)
1 cup, packed, fresh mint, coarsely chopped
   (both leaves and tender stems, with tough stems discarded)
1/4 cup water
2 tbsp lemon juice
1/2 tsp ground cumin
1/2 tsp ground coriander
1/4 tsp salt (or to taste)
1 tsp sugar
Optional: 1 fresh serrano chili, seeded and minced

Directions

1. Add half of herbs, along with lemon juice and water, to food processor. Puree until consistency of smooth paste
2. Add remaining herbs and ingredients and puree until smooth paste

Herb Tahini Sauce

The Basics: Blend
Yield: 8 servings | Prep time: 5 min | Cooking time: 2 min

Ingredients

1 garlic clove, pressed
1/2 cup parsley, coarsely chopped (both leaves and stems,
   with tough ends discarded)
1/2 cup mint, coarsely chopped (both leaves and tender
   stems, with tough stems discarded)
1/4 cup water
1/4 cup tahini
1/4 cup lemon juice
1/2 tsp salt (or to taste)
1 tsp sugar

Directions

1. Place all ingredients into food processor and blend
   until smooth

CHAPTER 33
SKIN SAVING SUPPERS

ROASTED SALMON ON ZOODLES

SALMON/MUSHROOM FRITTERS ON MIXED GREENS

ROASTED SHRIMP WITH TOMATOES AND ASPARAGUS

CHICKPEAS IN SPICED TOMATO SAUCE

I first realized how powerful a simple dinner could be during a lecture by an amazing speaker. Dr. Servan-Schreiber was the author of the book *Anti-Cancer: A New Way of Life*, and he came to speak at MD Anderson Cancer Center in Houston. *Anti-Cancer* is a great book, and it really inspired me to look deeper at all of the everyday ways I could improve our family's health.

In listening to him speak about the powerful benefits of spices, tomatoes, beans, onions, ginger, and garlic, I realized that I could easily start eating almost all of these ingredients in just one meal: my mother's chickpeas. After reading his book, I've since come across many recipes, from many cuisines, that highlight these and other powerful ingredients. In my home we tend to have certain dinners in our regular rotation, and I try to make sure that our mainstay dinners include these powerful ingredients.

This section is focused on lunch and dinner entrees. Many of the recipes in the other sections can take center stage for meals, whether that's a vegetable chili, quinoa salad, or spinach-feta frittata. This section adds a few other options.

Roasted Salmon: Omega-3s Salmon is an easy fish to cook, because its high fat content means it doesn't dry out as easily as other fish. Even better, those fats are omega-3s, and they're known for their powerful anti-inflammatory properties. The zucchini noodles add even extra flavor and nutrients.

Salmon/Mushroom Fritters: Power Fats and Carbs This recipe starts with salmon and adds in vitamin-rich sweet potatoes and mineral-rich mushrooms. These fritters do well on a bed of mixed greens, which adds in yet more nutrients.

Roasted Shrimp with Tomatoes and Asparagus: Lower-Calorie, High-Protein Shrimp is known for being a lower calorie, higher protein food. Roasting shrimp is an easy technique, and adding asparagus and tomatoes to the oven at the same time makes for easy cooking, along with a low calorie prebiotic food (asparagus) and a tasty, antioxidant rich food (tomatoes).

Chickpeas in Spiced Tomato Sauce: Rich in Antioxidants My mother, who's honed her skills in Indian cuisine over many years, taught me to make this chickpea dish. In Indian restaurants, you'll see different versions of this "chole" or "channa masala". This recipe starts with a mixture of cumin seeds, mustard seeds, and urad dal, then adds in onions, tomatoes, and more spices. Garam masala is a mixture of spices, and my mother prepares and grinds her own. It includes some of the strongest antioxidant spices studied, including cloves and cinnamon sticks.

I find it fascinating how traditional cuisines evolved   to maximize both flavor and nutrition. This recipe also includes turmeric, a powerful antioxidant and anti-inflammatory spice. Studies now show that curcumin, the potent phytonutrient present in turmeric, is better absorbed in the company of heat, fat, and black pepper.

Roasted Salmon on Zoodles

The Basics: Bake
Yield: 4 servings | Prep time: 10 min | Cooking time: 15 min

Ingredients
1 lb salmon fillets
1/2 tsp salt (or to taste)
1/4 tsp pepper (or to taste)

Zoodles (Zucchini Noodles)
3 medium zucchini, spiralized
1 tbsp extra virgin olive oil

Directions

1. Preheat oven to 400°
2. Season salmon with salt and pepper and place on roasting pan with skin side down (for easier clean up, line pan with foil)
3. Cook until salmon is opaque and flakes easily with a fork, about 15 minutes, more or less depending on thickness of salmon fillets. The general rule of thumb is about 10 minutes for every inch of thickness.
4. While salmon is cooking, heat olive oil in large skillet over medium heat
5. Cook zucchini noodles to your desired consistency, about 3-5 minutes
6. Serve salmon on bed of zoodles

Cooking notes: While you can purchase spiralized zucchini, there are several tools that can easily do the same at home. I prefer my inexpensive "pencil sharpener for vegetables". I use it the same way I do a pencil sharpener: insert zucchini, and sharpen.

Salmon and Mushroom Fritters

The Basics: Cook in skillet
Yield: 4 servings | Prep time: 10 min | Cooking time: 10 min

Ingredients

1 sweet potato, medium
1 packet cooked salmon, 5 ounces
Portobello mushrooms, 4 ounces, chopped
1/2 red bell pepper, diced
1/4 bunch cilantro, chopped (stems and leaves, tough ends discarded)
1 tsp paprika
1/4 tsp salt (or to taste)
2 eggs, beaten
2 tbsp olive oil

Directions

1. Cook sweet potato: wash, poke with fork several times, and microwave for 6 minutes
2. Once cooled, scoop out flesh and place in mixing bowl
3. Add all other ingredients (up to olive oil) and mix well
4. Form into patties
5. Heat olive oil on medium heat
6. Cook salmon cakes for 3 to 5 minutes on each side, until lightly browned
7. Serve on bed of mixed greens

Roasted Shrimp, Asparagus, and Tomatoes

The Basics: Mix and bake
Yield: 4 servings | Prep time: 10 min | Cooking time: 15 min

Ingredients

1 lb shrimp, peeled and deveined
1 tbsp olive oil
2 cloves garlic, minced
1 tsp each: dried basil and dried oregano
1/2 tsp salt
2 tbsp fresh chopped parsley, basil or oregano

For asparagus and tomatoes:

1 lb thin asparagus spears, tough edges snapped off (hold at both ends and bend until stem snaps)
1 lb cherry tomatoes
2 tbsp olive oil
1/2 tsp salt [or to taste]

Directions

1. Preheat oven to 400°
2. Gently combine shrimp and other ingredients in bowl
3. Transfer to baking sheet and arrange in single layer. (For easier clean up, may line with foil)
4. In separate bowl, combine asparagus, tomatoes, oil and salt
5. Transfer to a separate baking sheet and arrange in single layer. (For easier clean up, may line with foil)
6. Cook shrimp for 8-10 minutes, until cooked (pink and firm)
7. Cook asparagus and tomatoes until asparagus cooked, about 15 minutes depending on thickness of spears
8. Garnish with fresh chopped herbs

Chickpeas in Spiced Tomato Sauce

The Basics: Sauté and simmer
Yield: 8 servings | Prep time: 5 min | Cooking time: 30 min

Ingredients
Flavor base
2 tbsp olive oil
1 tsp each: cumin seeds, mustard seeds and (optional) white
urad dal
1 onion, diced
2 cans (8 oz each) tomato sauce

Spices
4 tsp garam masala
1 tsp salt
1 tsp turmeric
1/2 tsp chili powder

Main ingredients
2 cans (16 oz each) chickpeas, rinsed and drained (also
  known as garbanzo beans)

Topping
1/4 bunch cilantro, chopped (leaves and stems)

Directions

1. Heat oil on medium-high
2. Add cumin seeds, mustard seeds, and dhal. Cook until
   spices brown, stirring occasionally (about 2 minutes)
3. Add onion, tomato sauce, and remaining spices
4. Lower heat and simmer until tomato sauce thickens
   (about 10 minutes)
5. Add chickpeas and cover
6. Simmer for about 20 minutes, stirring occasionally
7. When ready to serve, add fresh chopped cilantro

CHAPTER 34
SKIN SAVING SIDES

ROASTED CAULIFLOWER

ROASTED BRUSSELS SPROUTS

RED LENTIL DHAL

HONEY GINGER ROASTED CARROTS

There are amazing chefs all over the world who are able to craft wonderful dishes centered on vegetables. I've seen vegetables transformed into intriguing appetizers, beautiful sides, or dramatic entrees taking center stage on the plate.

But it doesn't take much to transform vegetables, even in your home kitchen with simple techniques. These recipes utilize basic techniques: either the classic "shake and bake" technique or a simple "boil and garnish".

The Power Of Cruciferous Vegetables Cauliflower and Brussels sprouts are low-calorie, high-fiber, power-packed vegetables. That's just one of the likely reasons we're seeing so much of them on restaurant menus. (The other reason, of course, is taste.) Both are cruciferous vegetables, a group known for their potent health benefits. These vegetables contain organosulfur compounds. These phytochemicals are especially known for their ability to detoxify potentially harmful substances, as well as their anti-inflammatory abilities.

Both cauliflower and Brussels sprouts are also surprisingly good sources of vitamin C, one of the best-studied antioxidants in dermatology.

Roasted Cauliflower While cauliflower is considered a nutritional powerhouse, it can be a hard sell in its raw form due to its bitter overtones. One of the easiest ways to tame those flavors is to toss it in the oven. Roasting is a great technique for many of the cruciferous vegetables, since it mellows out the bitter overtones imparted by their organosulfur compounds. Roasted cauliflower has a mild flavor-even a touch sweet-and can be eaten straight from the pan or added straight to many other dishes.

Roasted Brussels Sprouts The same is true of Brussels sprouts-roasting does a great job of taming those bitter flavors.

Red Lentil Dhal: Fiber, Protein, and Phytonutrients Dhal is a traditional dish in India, and in some parts of India it's eaten almost daily. For such an easy-to-cook dish, dhal is exceptionally nutritious. With lentils, tomatoes, turmeric, and other spices, this particular version of dhal packs in a lot of fiber, protein, and phytonutrients. While lentils are fiber-packed and protein-rich, the turmeric and tomatoes also power up the nutrient profile. The addition of mustard seeds and cumin seeds in the "seasoning" adds even more.

If you've never cooked lentils, don't be intimidated: they're simple to cook. Just boil. There are different types of lentils. Some maintain their shape when cooked, while others, such as the red version used here, turn creamy.

Honey Ginger Roasted Carrots: Carotenoids This is another simple recipe that makes great use of carrots. Roasting carrots brings out their natural sweetness, making it an easy win flavor-wise. Carrots are known for their high concentration of beta-carotene (great for skin), and the ground ginger adds an extra flavor note along with extra nutrients.

Roasted Cauliflower

The Basics: Shake and bake
Yield: 6 servings | Prep time: 5 min | Cooking time: 25 min

Ingredients
1 head of cauliflower, chopped (florets and stalk)
1 tbsp olive oil

Spices
1/2 tsp dried basil
1/2 tsp dried oregano
1/4 tsp salt [or to taste]

Directions

1. Preheat oven to 450°
2. Place chopped cauliflower on roasting pan [for easier clean up, line with foil or parchment paper]
3. Drizzle olive oil, sprinkle on spices, and gently combine
4. Bake for 25 minutes

Cooking notes: This recipe tastes best when served fresh from the oven. Once cooked, you can add extra flavor by sprinkling on a few tablespoons of shredded Parmesan cheese and then placing back in the oven for 1-2 minutes to melt.

Roasted Brussels Sprouts

The Basics: Mix then bake
Yield: 6 servings | Prep time: 5 min | Cooking time: 20 min

Ingredients

Main Ingredients
1 lb Brussels sprouts

Flavorings
1 tbsp olive oil
1 tbsp balsamic vinegar
1 tbsp honey
1/4 tsp salt

Directions

1. Preheat oven to 400°
2. Slice individual sprouts in half. It's best to slice through the base, so that the base can keep the layers of the sprouts intact
3. Mix sprouts and flavorings together in a mixing bowl
4. Spread on roasting pan. For easier clean-up, line pan with aluminum foil or parchment paper.
5. Bake for 20-25 minutes.

Red Lentil Dhal

The Basics: Boil, then top with seasonings
Yield: 8 servings | Prep time: 5 min | Cooking time: 20 min

Ingredients

1 cup split red lentils (uncooked)
3 cups water
3 tomatoes, chopped
1 tsp turmeric
1/2 tsp salt (or to taste)

Directions

1. Add lentils, water, tomatoes, and turmeric to saucepan
2. Bring to boil, then simmer uncovered for 20 minutes
3. Add salt at end
4. When lentils are fully cooked, add seasoning (ask tarqa) for extra flavor and nutrients. See recipe on next page

Seasoning for Dhal (aka "tarqa")

The Basics: Cook in skillet
Yield: 8 servings | Prep time: 1 min | Cooking time: 5 min

Ingredients

2 tbsp olive oil
3/4 tsp cumin seeds
1/2 tsp mustard seeds
1 dried red chili, broke into large pieces
5-8 fresh curry leaves (optional)

Directions

1. Place oil, cumin seeds, and mustard seeds into skillet
2. Heat on medium-high
3. Stir occasionally until mustard seeds start to "pop", usually about 2-3 minutes. You'll need to watch closely, because the spices can burn quickly. (And watch out for flying mustard seeds.)
4. Add chili and curry leaves and stir for 1-2 minutes
5. Add to dhal and gently stir to combine

Honey Ginger Roasted Carrots

The Basics: Shake and bake
Yield: 8 servings | Prep time: 5 min | Cooking time: 25 min

Ingredients

1 lb sliced carrots
1 tbsp olive oil
2 tsp honey
1/2 tsp ground ginger
1/4 tsp salt
Mint leaves, fresh, for garnish

Directions

1. Preheat oven to 400°F
2. Mix all ingredients in bowl
   Place on roasting pan. May line pan with parchment paper for easier cleanup
3. Bake for 25 minutes
4. Garnish with fresh chopped mint

CHAPTER 35
SKIN SAVING SWEETS

PEACH/BLUEBERRY CRISP

PEACH ALMOND CUSTARD TART

FRUIT SKEWERS: STRAWBERRIES DRIZZLED WITH DARK
CHOCOLATE

OATMEAL BANANA CHIPPERS (GLUTEN-FREE)

I have a sweet tooth, which means I'm always searching for ways to satisfy that sweet tooth without doing too much harm. Desserts can do a lot of damage, and it can be a challenge to serve desserts that don't overdo it on the sugar and refined carbs. The following recipes provide a few options. While you still need to watch out for serving sizes with any desserts (these included), even dessert can provide an opportunity for some additional skin-saving benefits.

Note that all of these recipes make use of added sugar, although in limited amounts. If you're avoiding sugar completely, then skip over these, of course. But for many people, a small amount of added sugar is fine, as long as you're paying attention to how much you're consuming overall in your drinks, main meals, and desserts (these days, sugar is often added to all of these). I'm a big fan of making your own desserts, because you get to control exactly how much you're adding.

Recipes that center around fruit are a great place to start: they provide sweetness while still adding a boost of phytonutrients and fiber.

Peach Blueberry Crisp This recipe centers on peaches and blueberries, both of which provide antioxidant power. The topping of rolled oats and walnuts adds in an extra boost.

Peach Almond Tart The peaches in this custard tart provide a nice dose of vitamins, fiber, and phytonutrients. Using almond meal in place of white flour limits the amount of carbs, while eggs provide some extra protein to help limit sugar spikes. Finally, the sweetness of the peaches and the flavor from the extracts means that you can get away with less added sugar. There's only 1/4 cup of sugar added to the entire recipe.

Fruit Skewers This is a dessert that showcases the fruit, with a drizzle of dark chocolate adding in some extra antioxidants.

Oatmeal Banana Chippers For those who are avoiding gluten, these cookies have a boost of extra nutrients from the old-fashioned rolled oats, while using bananas in place of most of the sweetener helps to limit added sugar.

Peach Blueberry Crisp

The Basics: Mix topping then bake
Yield: 6 servings | Prep time: 5 min | Cooking time: 10 min

Ingredients

1 lb sliced peaches (fresh or frozen)
1/2 cup blueberries (fresh or frozen)
(if using frozen fruit, no need to thaw)

Topping

1/2 cup rolled oats (old-fashioned)
2 tbsp brown sugar
1 tsp cinnamon
1 tbsp coconut oil
2 tbsp chopped walnuts

Directions

1. Preheat oven to 400°
2. Arrange fruit in 8x8 baking dish
3. Mix topping ingredients together, and sprinkle on top
4. Bake for 10 minutes

Peach Almond Custard Tart

The Basics: Mix batter then bake
Yield: 6 servings | Prep time: 5 min | Cooking time: 30 min

Ingredients

Main ingredients
1 lb sliced peaches (fresh or frozen)

Wet ingredients
3 eggs, beaten
3/4 cup milk (dairy or non-dairy)
1 tsp vanilla extract
1/2 tsp almond extract

Dry ingredients
1/2 cup almond meal
1/4 cup sugar

Topping
Powdered sugar and 2 tbsp sliced almonds [optional]

Directions

1. Preheat oven to 400°
2. Spray pie pan with cooking spray
3. Scatter peaches on bottom of pie pan
4. Mix together wet ingredients
5. Mix together dry ingredients
6. Add wet ingredients to dry, and mix
7. Pour batter over peaches
8. Bake 30 minutes
9. Top with powdered sugar and sliced almonds and bake for 5 minutes more (optional)

Fruit Skewers

The Basics: Assemble
Yield: 6 servings | Prep time: 10 min | Cooking time: 5 min

Ingredients

1 lb strawberries, hulled
2 bananas, sliced
1 lb pineapple, chopped into large chunks

Topping

1/2 cup dark chocolate chips (at least 60% cacao)

Directions

1. Melt chocolate chips: place in microwave-safe bowl, and microwave for 30 seconds. Remove, stir, and continue to microwave at 30-second intervals until melted
2. Assemble skewers: thread strawberries and bananas on one set of skewers, with pineapple on another set
3. Drizzle melted chocolate over skewers and serve on platter

Cooking notes: Customize with any in-season fruit available. May sprinkle with chopped pistachios or shredded, unsweetened coconut

Oatmeal Banana Chippers
(Gluten-Free)
The Basics: Mix batter then bake
Yield: a/b 18 cookies | Prep time: 5 min | Cooking time: 10 min

Ingredients

Wet ingredients
2 tbsp coconut oil or vegetable oil
1 banana, ripe
1 egg, beaten

Dry ingredients
1/2 cup rolled oats (not instant)
1 1/2 cups almond meal
1/2 cup chocolate chips (60% cacao or higher)
2 tbsp sugar
1 tsp cinnamon

Directions

1. Preheat oven to 400°
2. Mix together wet ingredients in one bowl
3. Mix together dry ingredients in another bowl
4. Add wet ingredients to dry, and mix well
5. Drop onto lined cookie sheet
   (Lined with parchment paper or greased foil)
6. Bake for 10 minutes

REFERENCES AND ADDITIONAL READING

Included in this section are references, as well as some additional readings that you may find useful. Keep in mind that even with popular books, you still have to make sure that the recommendations apply to you. It's just like supplements: you have to think about the right supplement, at the right dose, for your particular medical condition. The same goes with dietary recommendations: whether it's related to the amount of carbs that you're consuming or the type of protein that's included in a recipe, you have to make sure that it fits with your medical profile, personal beliefs, and individual tastes.

Chapters 1-10

Fisher GJ, Kang S, Varani J, Bata-Csorgo Z, Wan Y, Datta S, Voorhees JJ. Mechanisms of Photoaging and Chronological Skin Aging. *Arch Dermatol* 2002; 138(11): 1462–1470.

Datta HS, Paramesh R. Trends in aging and skin care: Ayurvedic concepts. *J of Ayurveda and Integrative Medicine* 2010; 1(2):110-113.

Guruprasad KP, Dash S, Shivakumar MB, et al. Influence of *Amalaki Rasayana*on telomerase activity and telomere length in human blood mononuclear cells. *Journal of Ayurveda and Integrative Medicine* 2017; 8(2): 105-112.

Kabir Y, Seidel R, Mcknight B, Moy R. DNA Repair Enzymes: An Important Role in Skin Cancer Prevention and Reversal of Photodamage- A Review of the Literature. *J Drugs Dermatol* 2015; 14: 297-303

Katta R, Brown DN. Diet and skin cancer: The potential role of dietary antioxidants in nonmelanoma skin cancer prevention. *Journal of Skin Cancer* 2015 Oct 25; 2015.

Liu RH. Health benefits of fruit and vegetables are from additive and synergistic combinations of phytochemicals. *The American Journal of Clinical Nutrition* 2003 Sep 1; 78(3):517S-20S.

Liu RH. Potential synergy of phytochemicals in cancer prevention: mechanism of action. *The Journal of Nutrition* 2004 Dec 1; 134(12): 3479S-85S.

Melanson KJ, Greenberg AS, Ludwig DS, Saltzman E, Dallal GE, Roberts SB. Blood glucose and hormonal responses to small and large meals in healthy young and older women. *The Journals of Gerontology Series A: Biological Sciences and Medical Sciences* 1998 Jul 1; 53(4):B299-305.

Stutz M, Lawton GC. Effects of diet and antimicrobials on growth, feed efficiency, intestinal Clostridium perfringens, and ileal weight of broiler chicks. *Poultry Science* 1984 Oct 1; 63(10): 2036-42.

MORE READING:

Servan-Schreiber, D. (2009). *Anticancer: A New Way of Life.* New York, NY: Penguin Books: Extensively researched, yet very readable and practical book on cancer prevention and healthy lifestyles.

Greger M, Stone G. (2015). *How Not to Die: Discover the Foods Scientifically Proven to Prevent and Reverse Disease.* New York, New York: Flatiron Books: Very comprehensive yet easy to read and understand book on health promotion and disease prevention.

Pollan, M. (2009). *In Defense of Food: An Eater's Manifesto.* New York, NY: Penguin Group: Interesting and easy to follow book that discusses nutrition in a very approachable manner.

Buettner D. (2017). *The Blue Zones Solution: Eating and Living Like the World's Healthiest People.* Washington, DC: National Geographic Society: Highly recommended book focused on examples of communities living healthy, productive lives and the lessons learned.

Wansink B. (2006). *Mindless Eating: Why We Eat More Than We Think.* New York, NY: Bantam Dell: Humorous, enjoyable book focused on the forces all around us that encourage us to eat: highly recommended for those trying lose weight.

Chapter 5: SKIN SAVING FOODS

Bianco A, Buiarelli F, Cartoni G, Coccioli F, Jasionowska R, Margherita P. Phenol Explorer 3.6: A major update of the Phenol-Explorer database to incorporate new data values for lignans. *Journal of Separation Science* 2003; 26: 409-416.

Blando F, Gerardi C, Nicoletti I. Sour Cherry (*Prunus cerasus* L) Anthocyanins as Ingredients for Functional Foods. *Journal of Biomedicine and Biotechnology* 2004; 2004(5): 253-258.

Bonaventura P, Benedetti G, Albarède F, Miossec P. Zinc and its role in immunity and inflammation. *Autoimmunity Reviews* 2015 Apr 30; 14(4): 277-85.

Bourrie BC, Willing BP, Cotter PD. The Microbiota and Health Promoting Characteristics of the Fermented Beverage Kefir. *Front Microbiol* 2016 May 4; 7: 647.

Chen AC, Martin AJ, Choy B, Fernández-Peñas P, et al. A Phase 3 Randomized Trial of Nicotinamide for Skin-Cancer Chemoprevention. *N Engl J Med* 2015 Oct 22; 373(17): 1618-26.

Cosgrove MC, Franco OH, Granger SP, Murray PG, Mayes AE. Dietary nutrient intakes and skin-aging appearance among middle-aged American women. *Am J Clin Nutr* 2007 Oct; 86(4): 1225-31.

Croteau DL, de Souza-Pinto NC, Harboe C, Keijzers G, Zhang Y, Becker K, Sheng S, Bohr VA. DNA repair and the accumulation of oxidatively damaged DNA are affected by fruit intake in mice. Journals of Gerontology Series A: *Biomedical Sciences and Medical Sciences* 2010 Sep 16; 65(12): 1300-11.

Das I, Acharya A, Berry DL, Sen S, et al. Antioxidative effects of the spice cardamom against non-melanoma skin cancer by modulating nuclear factor erythroid-2-related factor 2 and NF-κB signalling pathways. *Br J Nutr* 2012 Sep 28; 108(6): 984-97.

Das S, Das J, Paul A, Samadder A, Khuda-Bukhsh AR. Apigenin, a bioactive flavonoid from Lycopodium clavatum, stimulates nucleotide excision repair genes to protect skin keratinocytes from ultraviolet B-induced reactive oxygen species and DNA damage. *J Acupunct Meridian Stud* 2013 Oct; 6(5): 252-62.

Dearlove RP, Greenspan P, Hartle DK, Swansen RB, Hargrove JL. Inhibition of protein glycation by extracts of culinary herbs and spices. *J Med Food* 2008; 11: 275-81.

Devarajan A, Mohanmarugaraja MK. A comprehensive review on Rasam: A South Indian traditional functional food. *Pharmacognosy Reviews* 2017 Jul; 11(22): 73.

Dog TL. A reason to season: the therapeutic benefits of spices and culinary herbs. *Explore: The Journal Of Science And Healing* 2006 Sep 1; 2(5): 446-9.

Draelos Z. Nutrition and enhancing youthful-appearing skin. *Clinics in Dermatol* 2010; 28: 400-408.

Du B, Bian Z, Xu B. Skin Health Promotion Effects of Natural Beta-Glucan Derived from Cereals and Microorganisms: A Review. *Phytotherapy Research* 2014 Feb 1; 28(2): 159-66.

Drewnowski A. Concept of a nutritious food: toward a nutrient density score. *Am J Clin Nutr* 2005 Oct; 82(4): 721-32.

Ejtahed HS, Mohtadi-Nia J, Homayouni-Rad A, Niafar M, Asghari-Jafarabadi M, Mofid V. Probiotic yogurt improves antioxidant status in type 2 diabetic patients. *Nutrition* 2012; 28(5): 539-543.

Fukushima Y, Takahashi Y, Hori Y, Kishimoto Y, et al. Skin photoprotection and consumption of coffee and polyphenols in healthy middle-aged Japanese females. *Int J Dermatol* 2015 Apr;54(4):410-8.

Ge Q, Chen L, Chen K. Treatment of Diabetes Mellitus Using iPS Cells and Spice Polyphenols. *Journal of Diabetes Research* 2017; 2017.

Giampieri F, Alvarez-Suarez JM, Mazzoni L, Forbes-Hernandez TY et al. Polyphenol-rich strawberry extract protects human dermal fibroblasts against hydrogen peroxide oxidative damage and improves mitochondrial functionality. *Molecules* 2014 Jun 11; 19(6): 7798-816.

Guo EL, Katta R. Diet and hair loss: effects of nutrient deficiency and supplement use. *Dermatology Practical & Conceptual* 2017 Jan; 7(1):1.

Heinrich, U., Neukam, K., Tronnier, H, Sies, H., & Stahl, W. (2006). Long-term ingestion of high flavanol cocoa provides photoprotection against UV-induced erythema and improves skin condition in women. *The Journal of Nutrition* 2006; 136(6): 1565–1569.

Imokawa G. Recent advances in characterizing biological mechanisms underlying UV-induced wrinkles: a pivotal role of fibrobrast-derived elastase. *Arch Dermatol Res* 2008 Apr; 300 Suppl 1 :S7-20.

Jy K, Ey C, Yh H, Yo S, Js H. Changes in Korean Adult Females' Intestinal Microbiota Resulting from Kimchi Intake. *J Nutr Food Sc* 2016(6): 486.

Kamal-Eldin A1, Moazzami A, Washi S. Sesame seed lignans: potent physiological modulators and possible ingredients in functional foods & nutraceuticals. *Recent Pat Food Nutr Agric* 2011 Jan; 3(1): 17-29.

Kano M, Masuoka N, Kaga, C, Sugimoto S, et al. Consecutive Intake of Fermented Milk Containing *Bifidobacterium breve* Strain Yakult and Galacto-oligosaccharides Benefits Skin Condition in Healthy Adult Women. *Biosci Microbiota Food Health* 2013; 32(1): 33–39.

Katiyar SK, Pal HC, Prasad R. Dietary proanthocyanidins prevent ultraviolet radiation-induced non-melanoma skin cancer through enhanced repair of damaged DNA-dependent activation of immune sensitivity. *Seminars in Cancer Biology* 2017 Oct; 46: 138-145.

Kim SR, Jung YR, An HJ, Kim DH, et al. Anti-wrinkle and anti-inflammatory effects of active garlic components and the inhibition of MMPs via NF-κB signaling. *PLoS One* 2013 Sep 16; 8(9): e73877.

Kook S, Kim GH, Choi K. The antidiabetic effect of onion and garlic in experimental diabetic rats: meta-analysis. *Journal of Medicinal Food* 2009 Jun 1; 12(3): 552-60.

Lee KK, Kim JH, Cho JJ, Choi JD. Inhibitory Effects of 150 Plant Extracts on Elastase Activity, and Their Anti-inflammatory Effects. *International Journal of Cosmetic Science* 1999 Apr 1; 21(2): 71-82.

Li D, Wang P, Luo Y, Zhao M, Chen F. Health benefits of anthocyanins and molecular mechanisms: Update from recent decade. *Crit Rev Food Sci Nutr* 2017 May 24; 57(8): 1729-1741.

Lim H, Kim HP. Inhibition of mammalian collagenase, matrix metalloproteinase-1, by naturally-occurring flavonoids. *Planta Med* 2007 Oct; 73(12): 1267-74.

Lorenzo Y, Azqueta A, Luna L, Bonilla F, Dominguez G, Collins AR. The carotenoid β-cryptoxanthin stimulates the repair of DNA oxidation damage in addition to acting as an antioxidant in human cells. *Carcinogenesis* 2008 Dec 4; 30(2): 308-14.

Moon NR, Kang S, Park S. Consumption of ellagic acid and dihydromyricetin synergistically protects against UV-B induced photoaging, possibly by activating both TGF-β1 and wnt signaling pathways. *J Photochem Photobiol B* 2017 Nov 7; 178: 92-100.

Nichols JA, Katiyar SK. Skin photoprotection by natural polyphenols: anti-inflammatory, antioxidant and DNA repair mechanisms. *Archives of Dermatological Research* 2010 Mar 1; 302(2): 71-83.

Oba C, Ohara H, Morifuji M, Ito K, Ichikawa S, Kawahata K, Koga J. Collagen hydrolysate intake improves the loss of epidermal barrier function and skin elasticity induced by UVB irradiation in hairless mice. *Photodermatology, Photoimmunology & Photomedicine* 2013 Aug 1; 29(4): 204-11.

Palombo P., Fabrizi G., Ruocco V., Ruocco E., Fluhr J., Roberts R., and Morganti P.: Beneficial long-term effects of combined oral/topical antioxidant treatment with the carotenoids lutein and zeaxanthin on human skin: a double-blind, placebo-control study. *Skin Pharmacol Physiol* 2007; 20: 199-210.

Perez-Jiminez J, Neveu V, Vos F, Scalbert A. Identification of the 100 richest dietary sources of polypheols: an application of the Phenol-Explorer database. *European Journal of Clinical Nutrition* 2010; 64: S112-S120.

Pérez-Sánchez A, Barrajón-Catalán E, Caturla N, Castillo J, et al. Protective effects of citrus and rosemary extracts on UV-induced damage in skin cell model and human volunteers. *J Photochem Photobiol* 2014 Jul 5; 136: 12-18.

Pittaway J.K., Robertson I.K., Ball M.J. Chickpeas may influence fatty acid and fiber intake in an ad libitum diet, leading to small improvements in serum lipid profile and glycemic control. *J Am Diet Assoc* 2008; 108: 1009–1013. doi:10.1016/j.jada.2008.03.009.

Purba MB, Krouis-Blazos A, Wattanapenpaiboon N, Lukito W, et al. Skin wrinkling: can food make a difference. *J Am Coll Nutrition* 2001; 20:71-80.

Riso P, Martini D, Møller P, Loft S, Bonacina G, Moro M, Porrini M. DNA damage and repair activity after broccoli intake in young healthy smokers. *Mutagenesis.* 2010 Aug 16; 25(6):595-602.

Roberts SB, Rosenberg I. Nutrition and aging: changes in the regulation of energy metabolism with aging. *Physiological Reviews* 2006 Apr 1; 86(2): 651-67.

Ronpirin C, Pattarachotanant N, Tencomnao T. Protective Effect of Mangifera indica Linn., Cocos nucifera Linn., and Averrhoa carambola Linn. Extracts against Ultraviolet B-Induced Damage in Human Keratinocytes. *Evid Based Complement Alternat Med* 2016; 2016:1684794.

Schagen SK, Zampeli VA, Makrantonaki E, Zouboulis CC. Discovering the link between nutrition and skin aging. *Dermato-endocrinology* 2012 Jul 1; 4(3): 298-307.

Shao X, Bai N, He K, Ho CT, et al. Apple polyphenols, phloretin and phloridzin: new trapping agents of reactive dicarbonyl spec *Chem Res Toxicol* 2008 Oct; 21(10):2042-50.

Shishehbor F, Mansoori A, Shirani F. Vinegar consumption can attenuate postprandial glucose and insulin responses; a systematic review and meta-analysis of clinical trials. *Diabetes Research and Clinical Practice* 2017; 127:1-9.

Sies H, Stahl W. Nutritional protection against skin damage from sunlight. *Annu Rev Nutr* 2004 Jul 14; 24:173-200.

Sim GS, Lee BC, Choo HS, Lee JW, et al. Structure activity relationship of antioxidative property of flavonoids and inhibitory effect on matrix metalloproteinase activity in UVA-irradiated human dermal fibroblast. *Arch Pharm Res* 2007 Mar; 30(3):290-8.

Sommerburg O, Keunen J, Bird A, van Kuijk FJGM. Fruits and vegetables that are sources for lutein and zeaxanthin: the macular pigment in human eyes. *The British Journal of Ophthalmology* 1998; 82(8):907-910.

Song JH, Bae EY, Choi G, Hyun JW, et al. Protective effect of mango (Mangifera indica L.) against UVB-induced skin aging in hairless mice. *Photodermatol Photoimmunol Photomed* 2013 Apr; 29(2):84-9.

Srinivasan K. Plant foods in the management of diabetes mellitus: spices as beneficial antidiabetic food adjuncts. *International Journal of Food Sciences and Nutrition* 2005 Jan 1; 56(6): 399-414.

Thring TS, Hili P, Naughton DP. Anti-collagenase, anti-elastase and anti-oxidant activities of extracts from 21 plants. *BMC Complementary and Alternative Medicine* 2009 Aug 4; 9(1): 27.

Trinidad TP, Valdez DH, Loyola AS, et al. Glycaemic index of different coconut (Cocos nucifera)-flour products in normal and diabetic subjects. *British Journal of Nutrition.* 2003;90(3):551-556.

Tsao R. Chemistry and Biochemistry of Dietary Polyphenols. *Nutrients* 2010; 2(12): 1231-1246.

Uribarri J, Woodruff S, Goodman S, Cai W, Chen X, Pyzik R, Yong A, Striker GE, Vlassara H. Advanced glycation end products in foods and a practical guide to their reduction in the diet. *Journal of the American Dietetic Association* 2010 Jun 30; 110(6):911-6.

USDA/Agricultural Research Service. Luteolin stars in study of healthful plant compounds. ScienceDaily. https://www.sciencedaily.com/releases/2010/07/100708141622.htm. Published July 16, 2010. Accessed December 21, 2017.

Vardy JL, Kricker A, St. George G. A phase 3 randomized trial of nicotinamide for skin-cancer chemoprevention. *New England Journal of Medicine* 2015 Oct 22; 373(17): 1618-26.

Vaughn AR, Branum A, Sivamani RK. Effects of Turmeric (Curcuma longa) on Skin Health: A Systematic Review of the Clinical Evidence. *Phytother Res* 2016; 30: 1243-64.

Wallace TC, Murray R, Zelman KM. The Nutritional Value and Health Benefits of Chickpeas and Hummus. *Nutrients* 2016; 8(12):766.

Watzl B, Kulling SE, Möseneder J, Barth SW, Bub A. A 4-wk intervention with high intake of carotenoid-rich vegetables and fruit reduces plasma C-reactive protein in healthy, nonsmoking men. *Am J Clin Nutr* 2005; 82: 1052–8.

Weh WJ, Jsia SM, Lee WH, Wu CH. Polyphenols with antiglycation activity and mechanisms of action: A review of recent findings. *J Food Drug Anal* 2017 Jan; 25(1): 84-92.

Weiss DJ, Anderton CR. Determination of catechins in matcha green tea by micellar electrokinetic chromatography. *J Chromatogr A* 2003 Sep 5; 1011(1-2): 173-80.

Whitehead RD, Re D, Xiao D, Ozakinci G, Perrett DI. You are what you eat: Within-subject increases in fruit and vegetable consumption confer beneficial skin-color changes. *PloS One* 2012 Mar 7; 7(3): e32988.

Yan M, Liu Z, Yang H, Li C, Chen H, Liu Y, Zhao M, Zhu Y. Luteolin decreases the UVA-induced autophagy of human skin fibroblasts by scavenging ROS. *Molecular Medicine Reports* 2016 Sep 1; 14(3): 1986-92.

Chapter 11: THE LAWS OF MEDICINE AND NUTRITION

Dao MC, Everard A, Aron-Wisnewsky J, Sokolovska N, et al. Akkermansia muciniphila and improved metabolic health during a dietary intervention in obesity: relationship with gut microbiome richness and ecology. *Gut* 2015; 22: 2014.

Melanson KJ, Greenberg AS, Ludwig DS, Saltzman E, Dallal GE, Roberts SB. Blood glucose and hormonal responses to small and large meals in healthy young and older women. *The Journals of Gerontology Series A: Biological Sciences and Medical Sciences* 1998 Jul 1; 53(4): B299-305.

Mullin GE. The good gut diet: turn your digestive system into a fat-Burning machine. Emmaus, PA: Rodale; 2015.

Qi L. Gene-diet interaction and weight loss. *Curr Opin Lipidol* 2014 Feb; 25(1): 27.

Zhang X, Qi Q, Zhang C, Smith SR, Hu FB, Sacks FM, Bray GA, Qi L. FTO Genotype and 2-Year Change in Body Composition and Fat Distribution in Response to Weight-Loss Diets. *Diabetes* 2012 Nov 1; 61(11): 3005-11.

Chapter 12: ANTIOXIDANTS

Carlsen MH, Halvorsen BL, Holte K, et al. The total antioxidant content of more than 3100 foods, beverages, spices, herbs and supplements used worldwide. *Nutrition Journal* 2010; 9: 3. doi:10.1186/1475-2891-9-3.

Halvorsen BL, Carlsen MH, Phillips KM, Bøhn SK, Holte K, Jacobs DR, Blomhoff R. Content of redox-active compounds (ie, antioxidants) in foods consumed in the United States. *The American Journal Of Clinical Nutrition* 2006 Jul 1; 84(1): 95-135.

Liu R. Health-Promoting Components of Fruits and Vegetables in the Diet. *Adv Nutr* 2013 May; 4(3): 384S–392S.

Chapter 13: INFLAMMATION

Buckley DI, Fu R, Freeman M, Rogers K, Helfand M. C-reactive protein as a risk factor for coronary heart disease: a systematic review and meta-analyses for the US Preventive Services Task Force. *Annals of Internal Medicine* 2009 Oct 6; 151(7): 483-95.

Curb JD, Abbott RD, Rodriguez BL, Sakkinen P, Popper JS, Yano K, Tracy RP. C-reactive protein and the future risk of thromboembolic stroke in healthy men. *Circulation* 2003 Apr 22; 107(15): 2016-20.

Harmon BE, Wirth MD, Boushey CJ, Wilkens LR, et al. The Dietary Inflammatory Index Is Associated with Colorectal Cancer Risk in the Multiethnic Cohort. *The Journal of Nutrition* 2017 Mar 1; 147(3): 430-8.

Koyama A, O'Brien J, Weuve J, Blacker D, Metti AL, Yaffe K. The role of peripheral inflammatory markers in dementia and Alzheimer's disease: a meta-analysis. *Journals of Gerontology Series A: Biomedical Sciences and Medical Sciences* 2012 Sep 14; 68(4): 433-40.

Shivappa N, Steck SE, Hurley TG, Hussey JR, Hébert JR. Designing and developing a literature-derived, population-based dietary inflammatory index. *Public Health Nutrition* 2014 Aug; 17(8): 1689-96.

Chapter 14: HERBS AND SPICES:

Aggarwal BB, Shishodia S. Suppression of the Nuclear Factor-κB Activation Pathway by Spice-Derived Phytochemicals: Reasoning for Seasoning. *Annals of the New York Academy of Sciences* 2004 Dec 1; 1030(1): 434-41.

Aggarwal BB, Yuan W, Li S, Gupta SC. Curcumin-free turmeric exhibits anti-inflammatory and anticancer activities: Identification of novel components of turmeric. *Molecular Nutrition & Food Research* 2013 Sep 1; 57(9): 1529-42.

Allen RW, Schwartzman E, Baker WL, Coleman CI, Phung OJ. Cinnamon use in type 2 diabetes: an updated systematic review and meta-analysis. *Annals of Family Medicine* 2013 Sep 1; 11(5): 452-9.

Kaefer CM, Miler JA. The role of herbs and spices in cancer prevention. *J Nutr Biochem* 2008 Jun; 19(6): 347-61.

Neelakantan N, Narayanan M, de Souza RJ, van Dam RM. Effect of fenugreek (Trigonella foenum-graecum L.) intake on glycemia: a meta-analysis of clinical trials. *Nutrition Journal* 2014 Jan 18; 13(1): 7.

San Chang J, Wang KC, Yeh CF, Shieh DE, Chiang LC. Fresh ginger (Zingiber officinale) has anti-viral activity against human respiratory syncytial virus in human respiratory tract cell lines. *Journal of Ethnopharmacology* 2013 Jan 9; 145(1): 146-51.

Saraswat M, Reddy PY, Muthenna P, Reddy GB. Prevention of non-enzymic glycation of proteins by dietary agents: prospects for alleviating diabetic complications. *British Journal of Nutrition* 2008 Nov; 101(11): 1714-21.

Shan B, Cai T, Sun M, Corke H. Antioxidant Capacity of 26 Spice Extracts and Characterization of Their Phenolic Constituents. *Journal of Agricultural and Food Chemistry* 2005: 53: 7749-7759.

Srinivasan K. Plant foods in the management of diabetes mellitus: spices as beneficial antidiabetic food adjuncts. *International Journal of Food Sciences and Nutrition* 2005 Jan 1; 56(6): 399-414.

Yashin A, Yashin Y, Xia X, Nemzer B. Antioxidant Activity of Spices and Their Impact on Human Health: A Review. *Antioxidants* (Basel) 2017 Sep 15; 6(3).

MORE READING:

Aggarwal B, Yost D. (2011 *Healing Spices: How to Use 50 Everyday and Exotic Spices to Boost Health and Beat Disease*. New York, NY: Sterling: A comprehensive, easy to read and understand guide to herbs and spices, with recipes included.

Chapter 15: POWER CARBS:

Karl JP, Meydani M, Barnett JB, Vanegas SM, et al. Substituting whole grains for refined grains in a 6-wk randomized trial favorably affects energy-balance metrics in healthy men and postmenopausal women. *Am J Clin Nutr* 2017 Mar; 105(3): 589-599.

The Nutrition Source. (2018). *Whole Grains*. [online] Available at: https://www.hsph.harvard.edu/nutritionsource/whole-grains/ [Accessed 22 Jan. 2018].

Chapter 16: POWER FATS:

Black HS, Thornby JI, Gerguis J, Lenger W. Influence of dietary omega-6, -3 fatty acid sources on the initiation and promotion stages of photocarcinogenesis. *Photochem Photobiol* 1992; 56: 195-99.

Boelsma E, Hendriks HF, Roza L. Nutritional skin care: health effects of micronutrients and fatty acids. *The American Journal of Clinical Nutrition* 2001; 73(5): 853-64.

Finch J, Munhutu MN, Whitaker-Worth DL. Atopic dermatitis and nutrition. *Clin Dermatol* 2010; 28(6): 605–14.

Latreille J, Kesse-Guyot E, Malvy D, Andreeva V, Galan P, Tschachler E, et al. (2012) Dietary Monounsaturated Fatty Acids Intake and Risk of Skin Photoaging. *PLoS ONE* 7(9): e44490.

Nagata C, Nakamura K, Wada K, Oba S, Hayashi M, et al. (2010) Association of dietary fat, vegetables and antioxidant micronutrients with skin aging in Japanese women. *Br J Nutr* 103: 1493 –1498.

Rhodes LE, O'Farrell S, Jackson MJ, Friedmann PS. 1994. Dietary fish-oil supplementation in humans reduces UVBerythemal sensitivity but increases epidermal lipid peroxidation. *Invest. Dermatol* 103: 151-54.

Rhodes LE, Shahbakhti H, Azurdia RM, Moison RM, Steenwinkel MJ, et al. 2003. Effect of eicosapentaenoic acid, an omega-3 polyunsaturated fatty acid, on UVR-related cancer risk in humans. An assessment of early genotoxic markers. *Carcinogenesis* 24: 919-25.

U.S. Department of Health and Human Services and U.S. Department of Agriculture. *2015–2020 Dietary Guidelines for Americans*. 8th Edition. December 2015.

Chapter 17: PREBIOTICS AND PROBIOTICS:

Chang YS, Trivedi MK, Jha A, Lin YF, Dimaano L, Garcia-Romero MT. Synbiotics for prevention and treatment of atopic dermatitis: a meta-analysis of randomized clinical trials. *JAMA Pediatr* 2016;170(3): 236–42.

Gibson GR, Scott KP, Rastall RA, Tuohy KM, Hotchkiss A, Dubert-Ferrandon A, Gareau M, Murphy EF, Saulnier D, Loh G. Dietary prebiotics: current status and new definition. *Food Sci Technol Bull Funct Foods* 2010; 7: 1-19.

Gueniche A., Phillippe D., Bastien P., Reuteler G., Blum S., Castiel-Higounenc I. Randomised double-blind placebo-controlled study of the effect of Lactobacillus paracasei NCC 2461 on skin reactivity. *Benef Microbes* 2014; 5: 137–145.

Hacini-Rachinel, F., Gheit, H., Le Luduec, J. B., Dif, F., Nancey, S., & Kaiserlian, D. (2009). Oral probiotic control skin inflammation by acting on both effector and regulatory T cells. *PLoS One* 2009; 4(3): e4903.

Heizer WD, Southern S, McGovern S. The role of diet in symptoms of irritable bowel syndrome in adults: a narrative review. *Journal of the American Dietetic Association* 2009 Jul 31; 109(7): 1204-14.

Hemarajata P, Versalovic J. Effects of probiotics on gut microbiota: mechanisms of intestinal immunomodulation and neuromodulation. *Ther Adv Gastro* 2013; 6(1): 39–51.

Holscher HD. Dietary fiber and prebiotics and the gastrointestinal microbiota *Gut Microbes* 2017; 8(2): 172–184.

Jensen G., Benson K., Carter S., Endres J. Ganeden BC30 cell wall and metabolites: anti-inflammatory and immune modulating effects in vitro. *BMC Immunol* 2010; 11: 15.

Picardo, M., & Ottaviani, M. (2014). Skin Microbiome and Skin Disease The Example of Rosacea, 48(December), 85–86.

Scourboutakos MJ, Franco-Arellano B, Murphy SA, Norsen S, Comelli EM, L'Abbe MR. Mismatch between Probiotic Benefits in Trials versus Food Products. *Nutrients* 2017 Apr; 9(4): 400.

Turnbaugh PJ, Ridaura VK, Faith JJ, Rey FE, Knight R, Gordon JI.The effect of diet on the human gut microbiome: a metagenomic analysis In humanized gnotobiotic mice. *Sci Transl Med* 2009 Nov 11; 1(6): 6-14.

MORE READING:

Mullin G. (2017). *The Gut Balance Revolution: Boost Your Metabolism, Restore Your Inner Ecology, and Lose the Weight for Good!* Emmaus, PA: Rodale: Very comprehensive, extensively referenced guide for those with gut dysbiosis.

Chutkan R. (2013). *Gutbliss: A 10-Day Plan to Ban Bloat, Flush Toxins, and Dump Your Digestive Baggage.* New York, NY: Penguin Group: Easy to read and understand.

Chapter 18: STOP SUGAR SPIKES:

Abid A, Ahmad S, Waheed A. Screening for Type II Diabetes Mellitus in the United States: The Present and the Future. Clinical medicine insights. *Endocrinology and Diabetes* 2016; 9: 19.

Akash MS, Rehman K, Chen S. Spice plant Allium cepa: Dietary supplement for treatment of type 2 diabetes mellitus. *Nutrition* 2014 Oct 31;30(10):1128-37.

Atkinson FS, Foster-Powell K, Brand-Miller JC. International tables of glycemic index and glycemic load values: 2008. *Diabetes Care* 2008 Dec 1; 31(12): 2281-3.

Caramel Frappuccino® Blended Coffee. Starbucks Coffee Company. https://www.starbucks.com/menu/drinks/frappuccino-blended-beverages/caramel-frappuccino-blended-beverage. Accessed December 13, 2017.

Centers for Disease Control and Prevention. National diabetes statistics report: estimates of diabetes and its burden in the United States, 2014. Atlanta, GA: US Department of Health and Human Services. 2014 Sep; 2014.

Dunstan DW, Kingwell BA, Larsen R, Healy GN, et al. Breaking up prolonged sitting reduces postprandial glucose and insulin responses. *Diabetes Care* 2012 May 1; 35(5): 976-83.

Ge Q, Chen L, Chen K. Treatment of Diabetes Mellitus Using iPS Cells and Spice Polyphenols. *Journal of Diabetes Research* 2017; 2017.

Gujral UP, Vittinghoff E, Mongraw-Chaffin M, Vaidya D, et al. Cardiometabolic Abnormalities Among Normal-Weight Persons From Five Racial/Ethnic Groups in the United States: A Cross-sectional Analysis of Two Cohort Studies Cardiometabolic Abnormalities Among Normal-Weight Persons. *Annals of Internal Medicine* 2017 May 2; 166(9): 628-36.

Healthy Eating Plate & Healthy Eating Pyramid. The Nutrition Source. https://www.hsph.harvard.edu/nutritionsource/healthy-eating-plate/. Published August 24, 2017. Accessed December 13, 2017.

Hernández-Alonso P, Salas-Salvadó J, Baldrich-Mora M, Juanola-Falgarona M, Bulló M. Beneficial effect of pistachio consumption on glucose metabolism, insulin resistance, inflammation, and related metabolic risk markers: a randomized clinical trial. *Diabetes Care* 2014 Nov 1; 37(11): 3098-105.

Johnson RK, Appel LJ, Brands M, Howard BV, et al. Dietary sugars intake and cardiovascular health. *Circulation* 2009 Sep 15; 120(11): 1011-20.

Kastorini CM, Panagiotakos DB. Dietary patterns and prevention of type 2 diabetes: from research to clinical practice; a systematic review. *Current Diabetes Reviews* 2009 Nov 1; 5(4): 221-7.

Khan A, Zaman G, Anderson RA. Bay leaves improve glucose and lipid profile of people with type 2 diabetes. *Journal of Clinical Biochemistry and Nutrition* 2009; 44(1): 52-6.

Khandouzi N, Shidfar F, Rajab A, Rahideh T, Hosseini P, Taheri MM. The effects of ginger on fasting blood sugar, hemoglobin A1c, apolipoprotein

B, apolipoprotein AI and malondialdehyde in type 2 diabetic patients. *Iranian Journal of Pharmaceutical Research* 2015; 14(1):131.

Koschinsky T, He CJ, Mitsuhashi T, Bucala R, et al. Orally absorbed reactive glycation products (glycotoxins): an environmental risk factor in diabetic nephropathy. *Proceedings of the National Academy of Sciences* 1997 Jun 10; 94(12): 6474-9.

Manore MM. Exercise and the Institute of Medicine recommendations for nutrition. *Curr Sports Med Rep* 2005; 4(4):193-8.

Medagama AB. The glycaemic outcomes of Cinnamon, a review of the experimental evidence and clinical trials. *Nutrition Journal* 2015 Oct 16; 14(1): 108.

Muraki I, Imamura F, Manson JE, Hu FB, Willett WC, van Dam RM, Sun Q. Fruit consumption and risk of type 2 diabetes: results from three prospective longitudinal cohort studies. *BMJ* 2013 Aug 29; 347:f5001.

Östman E, Granfeldt Y, Persson L, Björck I. Vinegar supplementation lowers glucose and insulin responses and increases satiety after a bread meal in healthy subjects. *European Journal of Clinical Nutrition* 2005 Sep 1; 59(9): 983-8.

Noordam R, Gunn DA, Tomlin CC, Maier AB, et al. Leiden Longevity Study Group. High serum glucose levels are associated with a higher perceived age. *Age* 2013 Feb 1; 35(1):189-95.

Reynolds AN, Mann JI, Williams S, Venn BJ. Advice to walk after meals is more effective for lowering postprandial glycaemia in type 2 diabetes mellitus than advice that does not specify timing: a randomised crossover study. *Diabetologia* 2016 Dec 1; 59(12):2572-8.

Rosolova H, Mayer Jr O, Reaven G. Effect of variations in plasma magnesium concentration on resistance to insulin-mediated glucose disposal in nondiabetic subjects. *The Journal of Clinical Endocrinology & Metabolism* 1997 Nov 1; 82(11): 3783-5.

Shukla AP, Iliescu RG, Thomas CE, Aronne LJ. Food order has a significant impact on postprandial glucose and insulin levels. *Diabetes Care* 2015 Jul 1; 38(7): e98-9.

Via M. The Malnutrition of Obesity: Micronutrient Deficiencies That Promote Diabetes. *ISRN Endocrinology* 2012; 2012:103472. doi:10.5402/2012/103472.

Winham DM, Hutchins AM, Thompson SV. Glycemic Response to Black Beans and Chickpeas as Part of a Rice Meal: A Randomized Cross-Over Trial. *Nutrients* 2017 Oct 4; 9(10): 1095.

Zeevi D, Korem T, Zmora N, Israeli D, et al. Personalized nutrition by prediction of glycemic responses. *Cell* 2015 Nov 19; 163(5):1079-94.

Zhang DW, Fu M, Gao SH, Liu JL. Curcumin and diabetes: a systematic review. *Evidence-Based Complementary and Alternative Medicine* 2013 Nov 24; 2013.

MORE READING:

Wolf R. (2017). Wired to Eat: Turn Off Cravings, Rewire Your Appetite for Weight Loss, and Determine the Foods that Work for You. New York, NY: Harmony Books: Easy to read, with discussion of variable glycemic responses.

Ludwig D. (2016). Always Hungry?: Conquer Cravings, Retrain Your Fat Cells, and Lose Weight Permanently. New York, NY: Grand Central Publishing: Nice discussion of the science behind glucose and insulin responses, with dietary recommendations.

Chapter 19: STOP SKIN SABOTAGE

Barcelos RC, Vey LT, Segat HJ, Benvegnu DM, et al. Influence of trans fat on skin damage in first-generation rats exposed to UV radiation. *Photochem Photobiol* 2015 Mar-Apr; 91(2):424-30.

Nguyen HP, Katta R. Sugar Sag: Glycation and the Role of Diet in Aging Skin. *Skin Therapy Letter* 2015 Nov; 20(6):1-5.

Uribarri J, Woodruff S, Goodman S, Cai W, Chen X, Pyzik R, Yong A, Striker GE, Vlassara H. Advanced glycation end products in foods and a practical guide to their reduction in the diet. *Journal of the American Dietetic Association* 2010 Jun 30; 110(6):911-6.

Chapters 20-23: DIET AND DERMATOLOGY

Bowe WP, Joshi SS, Shalita AR. Diet and acne. *J Am Acad Dermatol* 2010; 63: 124-41.

Chang YS, Trivedi MK, Jha A, Lin YF, Dimaano L, Garcia-Romero MT. Synbiotics for prevention and treatment of atopic dermatitis: a meta-analysis of randomized clinical trials. *JAMA Pediatr* 2016;170(3): 236–42.

Katta R, Desai SP. Diet and dermatology: the role of dietary intervention in skin disease. *The Journal of Clinical and Aesthetic Dermatology* 2014 Jul; 7(7): 46.

Katta R, Schlichte M. Diet and dermatitis: food triggers. *The Journal of Clinical and Aesthetic Dermatology* 2014 Mar; 7(3): 30.

Kwon HH, Yoon JY, Hong JS, et al. Clinical and histological effect of a low glycaemic load diet in treatment of acne vulgaris in Korean patients: a randomized, controlled trial. *Acta Derm Venereol* 2012; 92(3):241–246.

Schlichte MJ, Vandersall A, Katta R. Diet and eczema: a review of dietary supplements for the treatment of atopic dermatitis. *Dermatology Practical & Conceptual* 2016 Jul; 6(3): 23.

Smith RN, Braue A, Varigos GA, Mann NJ. The effect of a low glycemic load diet on acne vulgaris and the fatty acid composition of skin surface triglycerides. *J Dermatol Sci* 2008; 50(1): 41–52.

Smith RN, Mann NJ, Braue A, Mäkeläinen H, Varigos GA. The effect of a high-protein, low glycemic-load diet versus a conventional, high glycemic-load diet on biochemical parameters associated with acne vulgaris: a randomized, investigator-masked, controlled trial. *J Am Acad Dermatol* 2007 Aug; 57(2): 247-56.

Smith RN, Mann NJ, Makelainen H, Roper J, Braue A, Varigos GA. A pilot study to determine the short-term effects of a low glycemic load diet on hormonal markers of acne: a nonrandomized, parallel, controlled feeding trial. *Mol Nutr Food Res* 2008; 52: 718–26.

Weiss E, Katta R. Diet and rosacea: the role of dietary change in the management of rosacea. *Dermatology Practical & Conceptual* 2017 Oct; 7(4): 31.

MORE READING:

Website of the American Academy of Dermatology www.aad.org: Information on dermatology conditions

www.SkinAndDiet.com: Links to medical journal articles on skin conditions and diet, as well as regular blog updates on skin and diet

Chapter 24: MORE RESEARCH NEEDED

Barr S, Wright J. Postprandial energy expenditure in whole-food and processed-food meals: implications for daily energy expenditure. *Food Nutr Res* 2010; 54: 10.3402.

Chapter 26: LIFESTYLE AND DERMATOLOGY

Altemus M, Rao B, Dhabhar F S, Ding W, Granstein R D. Stress-induced changes in skin barrier function in healthy women. *J Invest. Dermatol* 2001; 117 (2): 309–317.

Axelsson J, Sundelin T, Ingre M, Van Someren EJW, Olsson A, Lekander M. Beauty sleep: experimental study on the perceived health and attractiveness of sleep deprived people. *BMJ* 2010; 341:c6614.

Chen Y, Lyga J. Brain-skin connection: stress, inflammation and skin aging. *Inflammation & Allergy-Drug Targets* 2014 Jun 1; 13(3):177-90.

Chiu A, Chon SY, Kimball AB. The response of skin disease to stress: changes in the severity of acne vulgaris as affected by examination stress. *Archives of Dermatology* 2003 Jul 1; 139(7): 897-900.

Cohen R, Bavishi C, Rozanski A. Purpose in Life and Its Relationship to All-Cause Mortality and Cardiovascular Events: A Meta-Analysis. *Psychosom Med* 2016 Feb-Mar; 78(2): 122-33.

Crane JD, MacNeil LG, Lally JS, Ford RJ, et al. Exercise-stimulated interleukin-15 is controlled by AMPK and regulates skin metabolism and aging. *Aging Cell* 2015 Aug 1; 14(4): 625-34.

Dunn JH, Koo J. Psychological stress and skin aging: a review of possible mechanisms and potential therapies. *Dermatology Online Journal* 2013 Jan 1; 19(6).

Garg A, Chren M M, Sands L P, Matsui M S, Marenus K D, Feingold K R, Elias P M. Psychological stress perturbs epidermal permeability barrier homeostasis: implications for the pathogenesis of stress-associated skin disorders. *Arch Dermatol* 2001; 137 (1): 53–59.

Hampl JS, Hampl WS. Pellagra and the origin of a myth: evidence from European literature and folklore. *Journal of the Royal Society of Medicine* 1997 Nov; 90(11): 636-9.

Holt-Lunstad J, Smith TB, Layton JB. Social relationships and mortality risk: a meta-analytic review. *PLoS Medicine* 2010 Jul 27; 7(7):e1000316.

Kumari M, Badrick E, Ferrie J, Perski A, Marmot M, Chandola T. Self-reported sleep duration and sleep disturbance are independently associated with cortisol secretion in the Whitehall II study. *The Journal of Clinical Endocrinology & Metabolism* 2009 Dec; 94(12): 4801-9.

Mourya M, Mahajan AS, Singh NP, Jain AK. Effect of slow-and fast-breathing exercises on autonomic functions in patients with essential hypertension. *The Journal of Alternative and Complementary Medicine.* 2009 Jul 1; 15(7): 711-7.

Ochiai H, Ikei H, Song C, Kobayashi M, Takamatsu A, Miura T, Kagawa T, Li Q, Kumeda S, Imai M, Miyazaki Y. Physiological and psychological effects of forest therapy on middle-aged males with high-normal blood pressure. *International Journal of Environmental Research and Public Health* 2015 Feb 25; 12(3): 2532-42.

Oyetakin-White P, Koo B, Matsui M, Yarosh D, Fthenakis C, Cooper K, Baron E. In Effects of Sleep Quality on Skin Aging and Function. *J Invest Dermatol* 2013 May 1: S126.

Pressman SD, Matthews KA, Cohen S, Martire LM, Scheier M, Baum A, Schulz R. Association of enjoyable leisure activities with psychological and physical well-being. *Psychosomatic Medicine* 2009 Sep; 71(7): 725.

Sinha AN, Deepak D, Gusain VS. Assessment of the Effects of Pranayama/Alternate Nostril Breathing on the Parasympathetic Nervous System in Young Adults. *Journal of Clinical and Diagnostic Research* 2013; 7(5): 821-823.

Walburn J, Vedhara K, Hankins M, Rixon L, Weinman J. Psychological stress and wound healing in humans: a systematic review and meta-analysis. *J Psychosom Res* 2009; 67 (3): 253–271.

Yosipovitch G, Tang M, Dawn AG, Chen M, Goh CL, Chan YH, Seng LF. Study of psychological stress, sebum production and acne vulgaris in adolescents. *Acta Dermato-venereologica* 2007 Mar 15; 87(2): 135-9.

Chapters 27-35: RECIPES

Jenkins DJA, Kendall CWC, Augustin LSA, Mitchell S, et al. Effect of Legumes as Part of a Low Glycemic Index Diet on Glycemic Control and Cardiovascular Risk Factors in Type 2 Diabetes Mellitus A Randomized Controlled Trial. *Arch Intern Med* 2012; 172(21): 1653–1660.

Wallace T, Murray R, Zelman K. The nutritional value and health benefits of chickpeas and hummus. *Nutrients* 2016; 8: 766.

Wang Z, Huang MT, Lou YR, Xie JG, et al. Inhibitory Effects of Black Tea, Green Tea, Decaffeinated Black Tea, and Decaffeinated Green Tea on Ultraviolet B Light-induced Skin Carcinogenesis in 7,12-Dimethylbenzanthracene-initiated SKH-1 Mice. *Cancer Res* 1994; 54: 3428-3435

MORE READING:

Bittman M. (2008). *How to Cook Everything*. Hoboken, NJ: John Wiley & Sons, Inc.: One of the ultimate guides for learning how to cook, and extremely comprehensive.

Culinary Institute of America. (2013. *Techniques of Healthy Cooking*. Hoboken, NJ: John Wiley & Sons, Inc.: A great resource for those interested in healthy cooking, with beautiful illustrations and instructions.

Kshirsagar A. (2011). *Smorgasbord of Indian Recipes.* Parker, CO: Outskirts Press.: For authentic and easy-to-follow Indian recipes.

Ramineni S. (2010). *Entice with Spice.* North Claredon, VT: Tuttle Publishing: A well-illustrated book on Indian cooking adapted for American kitchens.

Batra N. (2002). *1000 Indian Recipes.* New York, NY: Wiley Publishing, Inc.: A very comprehensive guide to recipes from many different regions of India.

Weil A, Fox S, Stebner M. (2014). *True Food: Seasonal, Sustainable, Simple, Pure.* Boston, MA: Little, Brown and Company: A cookbook focused on healthy and tasty food by Dr. Weill, who has written extensively in other books and columns on anti-inflammatory diets.

ACKNOWLEDGMENTS

Thank you to my mother Swarajyalakshmi Katta for contributing multiple recipes for this book. She has honed her skills over years of dedicated practice, and has always been so generous with her time and culinary wisdom and her unfailing support always.

I am very blessed to have a family who always go all in on my projects.

Thank you to my brother, Ravichand Katta, for being so generous with his all-around knowledge and help with my projects. Whether it's building a photography light box or finding the right piece of equipment, he's usually the first one we call.

Thank you to my sister-in-law, Anna Katta, who's a microbiologist and an amazing food stylist, and who's always willing to help out despite her very busy schedule.

Thank you to my brother, Praveen Katta, for being so generous with his photography knowledge and extensive skills, especially when he's traveled many, many miles to do so.

Thank you to my father, Satyanarayana Katta, for always volunteering to locate and obtain equipment and supplies for our multiple projects, and for providing unfailing support for years of projects.

Thank you to my nephews, Aleksander and Nikolas Katta, who are always willing to help out, whether that's moving boxes (ie furniture) or helping with the tech.

Thank you to my precious children, Shaan and Teja, and my wonderfully supportive husband and partner Samir, for contributing wherever needed and in so many ways, with love, whether that was cooking, washing dishes, designing infographics, food photography, website revisions, or teaching me the fine details of tech: what a talented team!

Thank you to my extended family, and family friends who are my family, for their consistent encouragement, support, and kindness, in Houston, Seattle, Detroit, Chicago, Austin, Washington DC, Richmond, Atlanta, Louisiana, Pittsburgh, Toronto, Ottawa, New Jersey, Dallas, Mumbai, and Andhra.

I have enjoyed many wonderful meals that have warmed me and inspired me. Thank you to all of the chefs who have fed me and shared their culinary wisdom, including my wonderful friends, my mother-in-law Suman Desai, my sister-in-law Poonam Desai, my brother-in-law Parag Desai, my cousins Neeraja Ketha, Biswani Kukkala, Shivani Tripathy,

Poonam Tripathy, and Nina Tripathy, and all of my warm, kind, supportive, wonderful Aunties.

And thank you to the next generation for feeding me with such care: Nikolas Katta (Andhra fish curry), Teja Desai (banana-oatmeal monkey bars), Shaan Desai (oatmeal chocolate chip chippers), Naya Desai (fruit salad), and Dilan Desai (lovely dinner companion).

I have learned from years of experience how much more we can accomplish with teams of talented individuals. I am very blessed myself to have worked with wonderful teams in running a clinic, in working on websites, in creating books, and in running a household. Thank you to my mother-in-law Suman Desai, my father-in-law Prakash Desai, my mother, my father, and Oralia Ramirez for providing the support needed to allow for a clinical practice and a book-writing career.

Thank you to my hard-working team for all of their contributions to this book and the website. Their contributions were very valuable and very much appreciated: Shaan Desai and Jasmine Nguyen on book design, Krishna Sigireddi on formatting, and Teja Desai, Sophia Huang, Jasmine Nguyen, Girija Shan, and Michelle Zhong on research.

I so admire the work of talented photographers, and am so grateful to these talented individuals for allowing me to use their work, and for their unfailing encouragement: Praveen Katta, Sharon Lunbeck, and Dr. Denise Metry.

Thank you to my very busy friends who provided such helpful reviews of early drafts of this work: Dr. Priya Ganju, Dr. Jodi Markus, and Dr. Jaya Reddy. It can be a challenge to provide supportive yet helpful feedback, and I so appreciate their taking the time to do so.

I have been very fortunate to have received the support and encouragement of wonderful dermatology and allergy friends and colleagues. I appreciate so much the work of the members of the Houston Dermatologic Society, the American Contact Dermatitis Society, and the American Academy of Dermatology.

During my 17 years at the Baylor College of Medicine and the Michael E. DeBakey VA Medical Center, I worked with wonderful colleagues, from the dermatologists to administrators to staff. A special thank you to the great team behind the Baylor Contact Dermatitis Clinic: Rita Agy, Tara Gray, Michaelynn Hughes, Sharon Lunbeck, Alicia Newton, and many others who worked so hard at the front desk, on the phones and behind the scenes.

Finally, I don't think we always realize the power provided by words of support and kindness and encouragement. A special thank you to our Aunties and Uncles and family friends who have always been so kind and encouraging, and to my friends who truly keep me going.

For More on Skin Saving Foods
and Research,
Please Visit

SkinAndDiet.com